ORANGUTAN BUTT-BURN DIET

Simple Eating, Health, and Exercise for Life

By R. Manolakas, MD

2

Copyright ©2015 by R. Manolakas

ISBN 13: 978-0-9898545-5-9

DEDICATION

This book is dedicated to everyone who is struggling to improve his or her health and quality of life. It's also dedicated to the endangered Great Apes of Asia and Africa (chimps, gorillas, orangutans), who are decimated by collectors, poachers, farmers, hunters, diseases, fetishists, and shrinking habitats. We must protect them before they are gone, which won't be long. Five dollars of every hundred in profit from the sale of this book will be donated to an appropriate organization dedicated to the rescue of these wonderful animals.

TABLE OF CONTENTS

ABOUT THE AUTHOR

R. Manolakas, MD, MBA, attended UC Berkeley,
UCLA, and the University of Nevada School of
Medicine and received his MBA from the University
of South Alabama. After years of clinical work, he
pursued a career in health management. He has
worked with the government and large insurers in
health care fraud and crime investigations. Dr.
Manolakas is Board Certified in Physical Medicine
and Rehabilitation—the medical specialty that
addresses body strength, mobility, endurance,
functional capacity, and illness, and is a past
Diplomat of the American Board of Pain Medicine.
He paints, writes, and is the author of three fiction
titles—all distributed under the quality Amazon
brands in Kindle, Audible audiobooks and I-Tunes,
and two paperbacks: *Subversion, Life on the Edge of
Eternity; Lonely Pines, A Medical Short Story
Wherein the Future Rescues the Past*; and *A Pool, A
Suitor, A Cellist: Bright Shadows Series, Novelette
Trilogies for Busy Folks*. He lives in coastal
California and is currently working on a medical
thriller novel series.

DISCLAIMER

As will be mentioned in many parts of this book, this material is not medical advice and is not intended to replace a work-up or review by appropriate, licensed physicians and trainers. Before any exercise or diet program is initiated, consult them.

INTRODUCTION

If you value your life highly, read this book and use its basic information as a blueprint for your health and vitality. Tweak it if you must, but use it.

Why diet and exercise like an *orangutan*? I like the catchy title—but it goes far beyond that. Orangutans, and other great apes, eat an abundance of vegetation and roughage and are not fussy how they do it. These creatures are constantly using their large muscle groups—the ones around their hips and shoulder joints—repetitively and intensively. They don't spend all their time checking their pulse and calculating calories and body fat—they just burn it!

Orangutans don't live in the past and the future—but the *present*. Anxiety is alien to them.

Furthermore, orangutans favor tree living, so they continually climb from branch to branch, equivalent to our activity of hiking. Their joints are extremely flexible.

In the wild, there are no fat orangutans. They don't smoke, binge drink, tailgate, or get hip replacements. Of note—especially to women who are bombarded with TV commercials about this—have you ever seen an orangutan with a fat ass?

I don't pretend to be an expert on apes, but I do know a thing or two about medical fitness, health care, and simple nutrition. So, it's humbly offered up here—with some common sense and a few tricks.

In this short and fast-reading book (that you can read in several hours), you'll learn to exercise and eat the way the orangutans would if they were human. Lady orangutans—I mean lady *humans*—will find this particularly beneficial, focusing on some of their special concerns. Hopefully, with some spicy humor thrown in (after all, I have to entertain too don't I?), you'll enjoy this book. However, my primary purpose is to *inform*.

I know—you've heard this before, with animal diets and time-consuming weight schemes by the hundreds. Nevertheless, if you follow this *simple plan*, it'll be most of what you need to reclaim your innate vitality and longevity.

Good health is not an end in itself, but the means to an end: enjoyment of life's bounty.

This book is *not* a replacement for good medical advice from your doctor. Although of great benefit to all age groups, its focus is primarily on the forty-plus age group. The kids are nearly out of the nest, you have your careers or social life established, you may have a few extra dollars and hours to spend, and degenerative diseases make their debut.

What follows doesn't target the morbidly obese, exercise fanatic, elite athletes, or, on the other side of the spectrum, people who just don't give a hoot about their looks, their weight, or their health.

This book is vital reading to the vast majority of average people (and generally middle aged) who must shed thirty to sixty pounds or so—and keep it off—and who want sound information as to how this will impact their medical care and the risk for some killer diseases.

The actual amount of weight to lose is dependent upon individual factors, and that must be discussed between you, your doctor, and your trainer.

First, the twenty-five to thirty pounds come off. Then, if you and your doctor agree, the second twenty-five or thirty come off. Then, you may want to make fitness your *hobby*—spend more time, money, and effort immersing yourself in the culture of fitness. Fine . . .

But, for now, it's a *battle*—a life or death struggle to many.

It can be fun too! When you finish the first level after six months, you'll be leaner, stronger, conditioned, and progress will be easier. You'll have a whole new life.

I don't have to go on about how fat our society has become and the extreme dangers that it poses. We all know that. Fly around the country and just watch the people in the airport or grocery stores and see how fat they are. See what they eat. It reminds me of the movie *Invasion of The Body Snatchers*, where near everyone is in the clutches of a powerful transforming evil.

One by one, we all succumb to the force of fat—but with this book—unlike the movie—you'll escape!

Weight loss is straightforward: calories *in* versus calories *out*, more or less.

You may refer to the FDA data on the nutritional content of food and daily requirements. We already have a good idea of those, really.

A juicy, one-pound steak is extremely high in fat, calories, sodium, cholesterol, and relatively low in fiber, compared to a pound of broccoli. That steak consumes a huge percentage of our daily allotment of fat, sodium, cholesterol, and calories.

As you age, it's almost impossible—in the real world—to achieve lasting weight loss if you regularly consume sizable portions of meat—and overload on starches. This is especially true with progressively sedentary lifestyles and decreasing metabolisms.

Although the author has a medical background, there are very few numbers and references in this work—and little jargon. Key sentences may have italicized keywords in parenthesis embedded within them, so you can Google the concept yourself for further study.

I've weeded out almost all the counting, measuring, journaling, weighing, calculating, and recording. With many weight control programs, you have so much of this you want to quit immediately!

Keep it simple.

The following paragraphs contain ideas you can remember and use. Each of the twelve brief chapters ends in take-home points, with Chapter 12 summarizing the dozen most important messages. Tear that off that twelve-point summary and paste it to your refrigerator, next to your favorite photograph of an orangutan!

At the end, you'll meet "Dr. Sheila Blue"—our fictional example of an overweight woman using the plan.

The photo will show a lean, happy, vibrant, and natural creature (absent a cellphone). That is what *you* want to be! While you're at it, read about their threatened survival (Google: *orangutan, photos, habitat, extinction, endangered, help*).

In our society, it's very difficult to avoid using brand names. I won't try. I receive *no* remuneration from any company mentioned in this book. I have no stock in them. I've used most of these products myself. Consider buying the machinery suggested in this book to best implement the concepts presented. In the long run, *you'll save money and time doing so*.

The aerobic (calorie burning) exercise need only take about twenty to thirty minutes per day—max—and the same with the progressive resistive exercises (simple "strength training"). Furthermore, take all the money you spend on *very expensive* gym memberships (although alternatively, you can do the exercises in your reasonably priced gym if you know how, and observe safety issues—24 Hour Fitness offers good value and convenience), plus pricy vitamins, meals, nutritional "supplements" (unless they're prescribed by your doctor), sport drinks, expensive groceries, other contraptions, and fancy gym clothes, and then invest the funds instead in the high quality devices that follow.

This book is the distillation of the author's experience and work with countless patients and clients in medical management, journal and textbook studies, and reading popular books.

Three excellent popular books stand out and acknowledgments are in order: *Fit or Fat* by Covert Bailey, *Body for Life* by Bill Phillips, and *The Vegetable Table: Thailand*, by Jacki Passmore.

This book does not profess strict vegetarianism (not a bad choice though)—but again—unless meat, starch, and alcohol is tightly controlled, there's much less chance you'll achieve the initial goal of a twenty-five to thirty pound weight reduction *in a healthy manner*—and *keep* it off.

The concepts contained here will, unlike "fad diets," be just as useful ten or twenty years from now. The food is simple and cost-effective—and in time, *tasty*.

Chapters 1, 3, 6, 8, 10, and 12 are the most important ones, and contain the majority of the vital information. But, read them all. They contain nuggets that help you cut through the maze of health care, doctors, and common diseases—many of the basic things you need to know to navigate away from the common killers that rob us of our vitality, productivity, and even our lives.

A major bonus of this book is to help you to dodge some of those diseases.

If you like this book, give one to your friend or spouse (do it together!). But to the guys out there—remember—always do your part of the simple cooking!

Good luck with your program.

Sincerely, R. Manolakas, MD; January 2015.

Chapter 1: Butt Burn and Calories

In this critical chapter, we will learn how to do aerobic conditioning so you obtain the most effective, efficient, sustainable, and safe calorie burn possible.

The key to burning enough calories is to repetitively exercise the big muscles in the major muscle groups that are used to working fast and hard. In other words, to use the butt muscles and the chest and shoulder muscles.

This means, of course, your "gluts" or the hip extensors, primarily. You want to isolate these muscles as much as you can and work them as intensively as you can to obtain an "aerobic benefit" that burns significant calories.

As I drive, I often see middle-aged people walking in the sweltering heat on the level sidewalks, teeth clenched and fists tightened, swinging their arms wildly in big sideways arcs, kicking their straight legs forward, leaning their bodies in grim determination. Although better than nothing, the time and effort invested could be much better directed.

These people are not exercising their gluts to capacity, but merely throwing their weight forward with their smaller muscle groups, with little hard metabolic work involved. If they are walking up steep hills, that's better, but this is seldom done.

Also, in elderly folks, heat puts a needless strain on the heart, and the sun exposes the skin to harmful rays. This walking on hard surfaces needlessly traumatizes the hip and knee joints—even when quality athletic shoes are used. Attacks from potentially vicious dogs and people (and fast cars with the pollution they bring) are also hazards.

If you enjoy the scenery outside, that's another thing, but that's not fitness—it is art.

Big muscle work, *focused*, is necessary to burn significant calories, and at sufficient *intensity* to induce conditioning. Conditioning leads to increased work capacity, and that leads to greater *marginal* increase in caloric burn and greater endurance. In other words, it's the fitness version of "the rich get richer."

How do you know your workout is getting more intense? First, your muscles will feel more fatigued, or will have a feeling of a pleasant burn—*not pain.* You will sweat more of course, your breathing will deepen or increase pace (but not too much!), and your pulse will quicken (if you check your pulse or use a pulse-meter you'll know for sure).

The pulse rhythm should be regular and not too fast!

You may also get a pleasant mental high if you exercise for long enough— or a general sense of wellbeing—this is an *endorphin* effect. These natural hormones are released during intense exercise and make us feel good.

You must remember that you have already discussed your program with your doctor and she may have suggested a target heart rate, and had set a maximum heart rate *not* to exceed.

If she did, you need a pulse meter (or to feel your pulse for checks). Discuss how to do this with your doctor or trainer.

If you have no medical *preclusions* to vigorous exercise (maybe after objective lab tests—see chapter 10), then you might enjoy your exercise more minus the hassle of taking your pulse frequently (without fear of a medical catastrophe). This is for your doctor and you to settle.

If your doctor's not interested (or trained in this), find one that is.

Many regard swimming as a wonderful form of aerobic exercise. It's certainly much better than nothing, especially lap kicking with short fins. However, for the average person who is not a formally trained swimmer, it's hard swim with the intensity necessary to burn large numbers of calories and to condition. It certainly is easy on the joints and pleasurable, assuming you have the time and access to a large pool.

Swimming is pleasant—but this is not fitness, it is art.

Ellipse machines are useful and easy on the joints. However, it may be very hard to maintain a neutral spine (a back posture that helps prevent injury—discuss that with your doctor and trainer). Much axial coordination and strength is required to do so.

Therefore, people of mature years should beware or they may induce or aggravate back pain. Also, isolating your gluts for intensive work may be more difficult than and therefore not as efficient as other forms of exercise that we'll cover.

Stair-climbers, while good for some, may not be the best choice either. Neutral spine and posture issues and a very real risk of falling may be problematic with this approach. Good balance is essential in utilizing this method. Therefore, the risk-reward ratio may not be as favorable as other forms of exercise—especially for the individual of mature years. The above machines are great, but for the right people.

Well then, just what *are* the best exercises to aerobically challenge the large muscle groups, and efficiently burn large numbers of calories and thus increase work capacity safely? There are indoor and outdoor choices.

First, the lesser alternative: outdoor. I love the outdoors for its open and airy feeling—but this notion is not fitness—it is art. Nevertheless, consider initiating a program of hiking safe trails if you have access to hills and slopes.

You may also walk various grades on sidewalks and the like (if the weather, terrain, and conditions allow). There must be hills. Wear good exercise shoes, socks, and loose, comfortable clothing. Wear a large hat to block harmful rays.

Jogging outside, especially for those of mature years, is not as good. Considering the trauma to joints and the amount of large muscle work expended per unit of time, it's inferior to brisk, graded incline walking.

Most joggers—especially the elderly—seem to throw their center of gravity forward with their smaller muscle groups, jarring and jiggling their bones, and don't selectively "burn their butts" or achieve the requisite intensity of selectively burning the largest muscle groups.

In outdoor activity with power-incline walking, start with a ten-minute brisk walk with progressively steeper grades of incline: level grade, 3 to 5 percent, and then maybe 10 to 12 to 15 percent.

Walk at speeds between 2 to 4.5 miles per hour or so, depending upon your fitness level, medical condition, size, and age. It will take you three to six months to achieve the upper part of this range.

Pay close attention as to how your muscles *feel* and how hard you breathe. You should strive for pleasant fatigue, but *not weakness* or *total* exhaustion. If you are walking with a friend, your exercise should not preclude you physically (due to labored breathing) from holding an easy conversation.

Make sure you are well hydrated. If you ever get dizzy or get funny pains in your arm or chest, stop and consult your physician right away (or emergency services!). You may start this program initially at three days per week, then work up to six days per week with a day of rest, adding another day of exercise every couple of weeks.

Gradually increase the proportion of high-grade minute walking within your ten-minute sessions. Your feeling of pleasant fatigue should guide you, knowing that you are exercising with adequate *intensity*. Since intensity is key, preferentially increase the incline before you add minutes.

If using a pulse meter (and your doctor may insist you do), you may also periodically monitor your target heart rate that you have established with your doctor and trainer, which may change with your conditioning level (*maximal heart rate, target heart rate, measure, exercise stress tests, aging, fitness, medical advice, safety*).

If you tolerate this exercise regimen adequately, then increase the number of minutes of each session by five minutes every couple of weeks, gradually reaching thirty-minute sessions. But first, again, make sure you increase your incline so that you achieve adequate intensity to ensure benefit. Intensity, not additional minutes, has the highest priority.

So, at the end of several months or so, whether it's walking on sidewalks or on trails, you'll be training with thirty-minute sessions, six days per week, with a day of rest. You'll have slowly increased your speeds and inclines—with steeper inclines your priority. During your sessions, it's good practice to start the first few minutes with low intensity as a warm-up, and finish with a few minutes low intensity as a cool-down.

A thirty-minute session, walked at 4 miles per hour with 12 to 15 percent incline grade—for 20 minutes (sandwiched between warm-up and cool-down), should offer a good selective "burn" of your glut muscles. This results in considerable aerobic conditioning and burning of calories.

This is more of a net benefit than *hours* of slow "flat-walking."

How do you know when you're walking at a certain grade, speed, or pulse level outdoors?

With experience, you gain a proximate idea naturally. However, there are commercial gadgets available (*inclinometers, pedometers, pulse meters, sale, fitness equipment, portable, training, measuring, speed*). For most, these will not be necessary.

Again, if you are cleared medically, you can just wing it, and estimate these things by *feel* and forget the hassle of measuring. Even if you're off by ten or twenty percent, so what if you don't hurt yourself and you are progressing?

Your doctor must clear you for this.

Ask your doctor.

To my mind, there are much easier ways to intensively and aerobically isolate and work your butt and other big muscles and get the caloric burn you need: "indoor" machines.

Remember, your goal is to concentrate on your big muscle groups for intensive work—which is the most efficient form of aerobic conditioning and caloric burn. These muscles have the built-in capacity to do steady work with less injury and fatigue.

Two machines that best meet this need: the reclined, variable-resistance and speed, exercise bike; and the wide, electronic treadmill with variable speed and incline controls.

First the treadmill: the good news is that you'll be walking and not running—so it's safer. The bad news is that you can still trip and fall (catching a toe), so be very careful.

This exercise is not recommended for very elderly folks with balance problems, or those who are careless. Discuss this choice with your doctor first. When using the machine, always wear the safety tether, which stops the machine in the case of a fall. If you can afford it, buy the wide version—it is easier and safer. Wear good athletic shoes that fit properly.

The routine is similar to outdoor hiking. Start with 10 minutes of walking, including a few minutes of warm-up and cool-down. In between, there are eight minutes or so of graded, inclined exercise at speeds that will provide enough intensity to burn significant calories and aerobically condition you. Make sure the intensity is adequate by preferentially increasing the incline degree and adjusting your posture.

Start at low levels of speed and incline, and gradually increase them over a few months. These speeds are generally between 2 and 4.5 miles per hour or so—depending upon age, size, and condition. Again, raise the incline level before your speed for the results we seek, because it offers greater intensity (and may be safer).

Be mindful of your back and neck, and try to use a neutral spine and proper posture to avoid injury or aggravation to an existing back condition. You must discuss this with your doctor first if you suffer from back disorders.

The variables with this machine are the percentage of incline, the number of minutes walking, and the speed of the treadmill. For safety and results, again, I think increasing the incline percentage and *then* the number of minutes is preferable, concentrating on your gluts, posture, and knee position to get the best *butt-burn* you can. *Feel* your butt!

Then, as you progress, increase the speed to safe limits.

I generally don't recommend over four miles per hour to avoid falls, and less for smaller and untrained individuals—and those who are elderly.

After several months (if you are cleared medically), you may be performing a thirty-minute routine six days per week, at 4 miles per hour and an incline of 12 to 15 percent, with 5 minutes of warm-up and 5 minutes of cool-down (where you walk slowly at zero grade.) This is only an example, and is dependent upon your individual case and your progress.

For this to work, your lower extremity joints need to be flexible and have adequate range of motion and strength. Prior to getting on the treadmill, proper, gentle stretching is indicated to avoid soft tissue injury. Your doctor or trainer may offer you advice in this regard.

Again, breathing, the pleasant burning (or slight ache or throb of your butt muscles—not pain!), your endorphin high, perspiration level, and your sense of pleasant fatigue will guide your intensity level. You can also use the pulse meter built into the machine to monitor intensity. Discuss with your doctor and trainer the pulse levels desired.

I think that reading (with the book holder), watching TV, and distracting yourself from your exercise is unwise and potentially dangerous. Be aware of what your body is doing in these short minutes and concentrate on your workout and the proper movement of your feet. Think about your butt.

Think about how much your butt is burning. Learn to feel the intense contractions of your butt muscles. Wearing headphones for your favorite music, however, can be stimulating and aid your program.

Ladies, if you want a tight butt, this, with general body weight reduction and proper nutrition, is a great way to get one. This anti-gravity exercise also loads your bones wonderfully, so it's excellent as a preventative measure against osteoporosis—a bonus especially for women.

There are many commercial treadmills to purchase for your home, and they have their own protocols. Any such protocol should be discussed with your doctor, trainer, and sales person. NordicTrack and Life-Fitness have machines that may suffice—check out several brands (*treadmill machines, exercise, incline training, aerobic conditioning, intensity*).

For the younger crowd who are already somewhat fit but not athletes or exercise hobbyists, an incline trainer treadmill is the most effective and efficient route to safely increase your aerobic capacity, conditioning, and calorie burn—and preserve your joints. The steep incline forces you to observe the principle of intensity, which, like other concepts, is repeated often throughout this book.

For the unfit and over forty or fifty crowd, however, we now come to my *favorite* machine— especially for mature ladies who prize convenience, safety, results, ease, comfort, enjoyment, and efficiency—with joint preservation. It's only slightly less effective than incline training if used properly, but not enough to be decisive. Intensity is available, but enforcing it is a bit more challenging than with the treadmill.

This wonderful machine is the electronic, reclined, exercise bicycle with easy, hand-controlled, variable resistance.

A padded, adjustable, sliding seat that puts your legs generally at the level of your heart is a plus, which slides back and forth to adjust knee and hip flexion and extension angles. It assists you in positioning for the maximum burn of your butt. Stirrups, which are easily adjustable and allow your feet to reposition properly on the pedal, are a must.

Several companies make such machines.

NordicTrack and Life-Fitness may be worth checking out (*exercise bicycles, reclined, electronic, conditioning, adjustable resistance, controls*).

The routine is familiar.

Ten minutes of exercise with a few minutes of warm-up and cool-down will be gradually increased to thirty, allowing your pulse (which the handles of the machine often measure automatically) and physical cues to guide your intensity. Increasing the resistance controls intensity, along with how fast you pedal. I suggest that you set a good speed (try 8 MPH) with your trainer, and then change the resistance to assure adequate intensity.

Buy the highest quality, longest lasting, and most expensive machine that you can afford—the investment will be well worth it.

Remember, as with all the exercises discussed, you simply must work at the intensity level that will burn significant calories and condition your targeted, large muscle groups to capacity, with a pleasant sense of fatigue or burn (but not pain). If you do not, your benefit and calorie burn will be *much less*.

As your muscles become conditioned, many people find that the sensation of burning, aching, or fatigue in the butt muscles becomes a pleasant one—and end up craving it. This is often accompanied by the "endorphin high."

It's best to position the feet in the stirrups so that the heels are driving the rotary force while cycling—not the balls of the feet. Pedal with the seat back so that the knees are between about 110 to 160 degrees through the rotation cycle—*to help facilitate a more selective butt-burn.*

Find out for yourself the best position to butt-burn. Shift your body around on the machine, concentrating on which position gives you the most intense use of the hip extensors—and which ones tax the quads as well (the knee extensor or thigh muscles). These are the large muscle groups.

The principle here is to have *wide enough extension angles in the hips and knees to selectively burn the butt.* Consult your trainer and sales person.

The beauty of this machine is that your hands, and your attention, are freed to allow you to read, watch a DVD or YouTube, use your smart phone, write, knit, roll cigarettes (just kidding!), or oil paint. However, consider just enjoying the burn! There's also minimal risk of falling, tripping, or significant back injury, with no jarring of bones or joints.

You may *also* exercise your *upper* extremity muscle groups at the same time!

Ladies, buy some five-pound dumbbells at Wal-Mart (guys, maybe ten-pound, depending upon what you and your doctor and trainer decide), and while you are sitting and pedaling, perform the following exercises: shoulder presses; shoulder "butterflies"; bicep curls; arm adductions for the "pecs" (bring your dumbbells together and apart over your chest); and triceps "reverse-curls".

Try typing some of these words into YouTube for guidance, and ask your trainer and physician how to best do these sitting exercises safely.

You might concentrate on the chest muscles, since these are the large muscles, and therefore burn more calories. However, the calories burned will be small compared to the sustained butt-burn.

As a bonus, you'll gain some upper extremity strength too (see Chapter 3 where the weight can be increased and the number of repetitions decreased to emphasize *strength* training rather than aerobic burn).

Perform dumbbell repetitions in enough numbers to obtain mild fatigue and the sense of burn (but not pain) that suggests adequate intensity and a modest aerobic conditioning benefit. The movements should always be smooth and not jerking, and not as fast as to be uncontrolled—to avoid shoulder, elbow, and wrist injury.

Again, consult your doctor and a fully credentialed trainer on how to perform these exercises (a good trainer is always a smart choice for *additional* advice—especially to get you started or to refresh your knowledge base).

There you have it, the reclined bicycle, and the inclined treadmill, for a sustained butt-burn from intense aerobic conditioning.

Intensity and butt-focus are the operative principals in this chapter, and exactly how you go about them is between you, your doctor, and your trainer consultant.

Take home points:

The indoor exercises are more efficient.

The reclined exercise bicycle is perhaps safer. Speed and resistance are the variables.

The incline treadmill is more effective, and, for ladies, better to prevent osteoporosis and to "tighten" the butt.

You may simultaneously work the upper body with the bike—but I think it's better to concentrate on your butt.

Pay attention to your posture on the treadmill to help prevent back injury or falls.

Position your feet and the seat on your bicycle to work the gluts most effectively.

Work up to a sustained burn of your hip muscles (butt-burn) with sufficient resistance to obtain fatigue and mild exhaustion.

Set progressive, graded exercise and pulse limits with your physician, plus any cardiac or joint preclusion *before* you start.

If allowed by your doctor, work up to thirty-minute sessions, with 5 minutes of warm-up and 5 minutes of cool-down, six days per week.

Hiking trails and walking sidewalks or other hard surfaces requires graded hills for the sustained intensity of your workout.

Remember, no intensity—little significant aerobic benefit.

The intensity of your workout can be estimated in subjective and objective ways.

Chapter 2: Easy on the Joints

By now, you have an effective blueprint to burn significant calories and to SAFELY and aerobically condition yourself.

Let's talk briefly about your joints.

The reclined exercise bicycle is the easiest on your joints and a great form of exercise to preserve joint function. If you already have bad joints, adjunctive exercise in a heated pool (which partially offsets the effects of gravity) is desirable to maintain range of motion and achieve some conditioning results, and to relieve some chronic pain conditions.

This is vital for the forty-to-fifty plus crowd.

Joint wear and tear, much like x-ray exposure and UV light exposure, is largely a cumulative phenomenon over life. We are generally born with only so much tread on our tires. Many of those folks who ran marathons on hard surfaces with mediocre running shoes in their twenties or thirties will face joint replacements in their sixties and seventies.

Save your joints and exercise smart.

Eliminate or limit bone and joint jarring activities, such as running on hard surfaces, tennis (although with proper technique in the social player this can be a good choice), handball, and the like. Another way to protect your joints is to make sure that the muscles around the joints are strong and conditioned—which is addressed in this book.

With proper exercise, your coordination and stamina is augmented, also protecting your joints.

You must wear good quality shoes that are appropriate for the activity in which you are engaged, with good heel cushioning and arch supports. A podiatrist can help you with that.

Weight reduction in itself is a great way to protect your joints. The ground reactive vectors on your weight bearing joints are much *less* (in a non-linear way) *with decreasing weight*, thus sparing your joints from needless wear and tear over the years.

You are on your way with this book.

Two common and major forms of diseases of the joints are *degenerative* and *inflammatory*—and at times both simultaneously. Degenerative arthritis primarily affects the large, weight bearing joints and advances with age.

An example of the inflammatory kind is rheumatoid arthritis. *Inflammatory osteoarthritis* is an example of both types—and is very common. It is vital that you consult a board certified rheumatologist or orthopedic surgeon to specifically address serious forms of these diseases, especially inflammatory arthritis.

There are specific treatments for inflammatory arthritic diseases—especially new drugs—that can help prevent joint destruction. Aside from avoiding the intense pain, you need healthy joints to exercise and to function!

So, get the help you need—there's no substitute.

Arthritis—including back and neck pain—is extremely common and can be painful and debilitating. Many cases improve no matter how you treat it. Therefore, there are zillions of treatments out there—good and bad. This includes both drugs and "dietary supplements." Many of these drugs are "over the counter" and so don't require a doctor's guidance. There may be less government oversight with the dietary supplements.

The efficacy of drugs and dietary supplements—and potential side effects—are best tested by randomized clinical trails with strict control groups, involving large numbers of patients and an independent funding source. Such medical studies, especially in this country, are getting fewer.

Many "clinical studies" are personal anecdotes, which carry little statistical significance. Many are poorly designed, with too many variables that cannot possibly be controlled—which effect outcomes. There is "expectation bias." Further discussion of this topic is way beyond the scope of this book, so just beware of medical claims.

Interestingly, one of the best methods to treat chronic pain (with the proper medical preclusions of course set by your physician) is appropriate exercise—especially that which generates the endorphin highs.

Also, beware of potentially harmful side effects of common mainline drugs, such as even generic acetaminophen, ibuprofen, and good old aspirin!

Taken *incorrectly* for inadequate reason, these drugs—in susceptible individuals—can complicate potentially fatal episodes of kidney and liver disease, gastrointestinal bleeding, and hemorrhagic stroke.

The manufacturers are the first to tell you this. Read the label! Consult your doctor.

Instead of hounding your doctor about prescription drugs pushed in TV commercials (and for which *we* end up paying), use any extra time with your physician to discuss your weight loss program and personal limits based upon your medical record (Chapter 10).

Take the money you spend on unproven or potentially harmful "remedies" not specifically recommended by your doctor, and put them instead in a fund for your new reclined exercise bicycle or deductibles and co-pays toward your health insurance plan.

The last concept in this chapter is the one that is most overlooked and hardest to correct—the loss of joint range of motion.

Aging, injury, and disease can change our joints so that the angles (or ranges through which they work) decrease markedly. This can happen even to the point of unsightly contractures or deformity of the joint. This may be caused by scarring of the soft tissue around the joint or by inflammation within the joint, which can cause pain and destruction of the cartilage and bone surface.

This causes the joint to be less functional and the muscles around it to be less efficient, working at a mechanical disadvantage.

Even in very subtle forms due to advancing age, this can seriously hinder our ability to exercise or perform essential tasks. Fatigue, pain, and restricted movement can defeat our conditioning efforts.

Therefore, gentle stretching exercises to all major muscle groups must be performed daily, even for just a minute or two. This is especially true for the hips. Consult your doctor and trainer for the proper stretches to perform safely.

You might also look up these exercises on YouTube and then discuss them with your doctor.

Take home points:

Discuss with your doctor and trainer strategies to protect your joints, and exercise smart; loose weight.

Chapter 3: Augment Strength

As we age, we usually get weaker. If we don't use our muscles, we also get weaker—at any age. Strength is necessary for good joint function and to perform activities of daily living. With advancing age and disuse (or misuse), our muscle fibers undergo atrophy—or shrink away.

Greatly advancing age and disease can bring "motor unit dropout"—or the dying out of motor units in our muscles. A motor unit is a clump of motor fibers enervated by a filament of nerve. A lot can go wrong with these units, and does—with some "dying off" or scarring down.

The good news is that nature had built redundancy into our muscular system—like other systems and organs—so the above may not matter much functionally. The most fascinating things about the human (healthy) body are its "redundancy," its resiliency, and its ability to rejuvenate itself.

All the supercomputers placed in series from here to China couldn't even begin to match the power and design of the human body. If we conclude that evolution is responsible for this miracle, one might also wonder: who made evolution? Well . . . just think about the power that the gift of the human body provides!

So, what does this mean?

It means that with proper training and conditioning, the motor fibers in your exercised muscle can start to grow bigger and stronger again—through hypertrophy—and other motor units will largely take over for the ones lost or weakened. For them to do this best, they need the right *kind* of exercise.

Which kind?

Yes, you got it—they need exercise that is *intense* enough.

Then, with growth they become stronger, more efficient, can sustain more force longer, and burn more calories per unit of time—often with a higher metabolic rate. This also consumes more calories.

It's the fitness equivalent of "the rich get richer" again.

So, just what exercises do we do to accomplish this?

Progressive resistive exercises are used for our strength training, carefully targeting the proper balance of the largest muscle groups for maximum results. This will also aid our caloric burn when using them in aerobic exercise by allowing them to perform more work (applied force) per unit of time expended short of failure.

This performance will be evident as we increase our work intensity in a graded manner over months with proper training.

What is the best form of progressive resistive exercise?

For the younger and more fit, so-called "closed chain" exercises—pull-ups and push-ups for example, can be very useful.

However, they can be quite difficult, take a lot of coordination and instruction on how to do them properly and safely, and offer difficulties in isolating certain large muscles. They may also require a lot of initial strength.

Weight training is—for most—the best form of strengthening exercises, especially for the elderly. This may seem counterintuitive, but it's hard to refute. Climate, resistance, range of motion of the joints, force, posture, and speed can all be generally controlled for maximum results and safety.

The two main types of weight training are "free weights," such as bars and dumbbells, and "cam" weights, such as Universal Gyms and the like. These are the contraptions with the pulleys and wheels in all the good clubs.

We've already discussed light, *free* weights in Chapter 1 in connection with aerobic conditioning and reclined exercise bicycles. Broader use of these can be very useful especially for younger, fit individuals who have been instructed in their use.

This type of weights runs a greater risk of injury because the weights are free ranging—therefore there is greater chance of dropping them, being pinned down, or exceeding your safe tolerance. This is especially true when using heavy weights.

The protocols for using these weights are similar to cam weights, the latter being preferable and will be discussed next.

Remember, if you choose free weights, consult your doctor and your trainer for clearance and proper use and posture (YouTube may also have some interesting demonstrations of their use—the same is true of cam weights).

For ease of intensity, again, "cam" weights are preferable. These are stacked weights on pulleys that adjust with pins. Lifting weights can be very boring for most, and so we must have a routine that encourages us to do our exercises and do them properly.

This is the key: it's much more important that you do them routinely and *intensively* rather than spending a lot of time with each session. You must do them right with adequate *intensity*. Spending time in endless sets of repetitions isn't recommended— because you risk boredom and socializing rather than focusing on intensity, with little gain.

You'll work the major muscle groups, including the all-important hip extensors, to the point that you feel a gentle burn, ache, or fatigue of your muscles (not pain). You also may feel a slight throb when you rest your muscle just after contraction.

You *must* concentrate on the muscles being worked. You must get a burn. You must.

You must contract your muscles slowly (about three seconds), and release even slower. Hold at the end of the contraction about a second. Exhale as you contract and inhale as you release. Always perform a minute or two of gentle stretches first, and always use good posture and a neutral spine to protect your back.

Consult with your doctor and trainer— especially initially—to be instructed in the proper use of the weights. Never jerk or slam the weights! That means that you are not using them properly. Many good health clubs have credentialed trainers right there—so use them, even if you have to pay. It is money well spent.

How much weight to use and how many repetitions (reps) should you do? This question generates controversy, and has become almost like an exercise management fetish. The best routine to use for our purposes is the "fifteen repetitions maximum" to fatigue, achieving a mild burn or throb—*not pain*.

For each muscle group, experiment with different weight loads so that you can perform only *one* contraction (safely) at maximum weight—in other words—it's hard to lift any more weight on that one contraction. Work with your trainer to avoid injury.

Then subtract about a third to a quarter of that weight and repeat the same contraction fifteen times *slowly*. After you complete this, you should feel like you can't do another rep. You should have a mild burn. Again, consider working with your trainer.

Your targeted muscles should feel a slight ache, burn, or fatigue. It's important to stop a few degrees short of complete extension or flexion (not the full range of motion) to protect your joints.

If you don't get that feeling of fatigue and mild burn, record the amount of weight and then add a little more weight the next time and then again until you *do* get that feeling. If it's too much weight and you feel discomfort *before* fifteen "reps," subtract a little weight and try again the next day. Titrate it until you arrive at the correct amount of weight.

Getting the burn with too *few* reps may not develop sufficient conditioning and optimal development of the muscles. Fifteen is a good number. Can I prove it is the *best* number? No, I can't. The important thing is that *each* rep should be slow and perfect.

When you find the right weight, stick with that weight for a few weeks with each muscle group.

The method is safe if done correctly, fast, keeps you from getting bored or running out of time, and is performed with sufficient intensity to get results: slight hypertrophy of the muscle with progressively increased strength and aerobic work capacity.

As bonuses, with general body weight *reduction* and a few months, you'll see increased definition of the muscles and reshaping of your body into a more visually pleasing form. For women, there is little fear of getting bulked up or looking too "manly"—so don't be too concerned.

For those who take anabolic steroids, that's another matter—and taking such substances is *not* recommended in this book unless it's under a doctor's order and for a legitimate reason.

Every few weeks you'll find that the muscle groups are no longer challenged (no burn) with the amount of weight you last selected, so gradually add a few more pounds to renew the challenge.

Progress will be forthcoming.

The muscle groups exercised will be: the deltoids (shoulders), "lats", the biceps and the triceps (arms), the pectoralis majors (chest), the quadriceps (front of thigh), the hamstrings (back of thigh), the calf muscles, the hip extensors (straight knee and bent—main butt muscles), hip abductors, and hip flexors.

Life-Fitness and others have excellent machines for this.

You may also add shallow, gentle abdominal "crunches" if you have no serious back conditions—consult your doctor and trainer.

Remember, you are doing it to the point of a gentle "burn"—but not pain. This is plenty to get you started, and you can always add some muscle groups later if you like. Exercising these muscles should take no longer than twenty to twenty-five minutes including gentle stretches.

I'd recommend earphones to listen to your favorite music, but no other distractions. Consult your trainer and doctor about prohibitions and preclusions, and to instruct you on the proper use of the weights—with demonstrations.

Again, YouTube may have some good video demonstrations. Your club trainers can be very helpful and convenient. Again, for the ladies, isolating the hip extensors with this form of exercise—with the general weight reduction and aerobic conditioning already discussed—will help sculpt the butt into the pleasing shape you desire (ok, guys too!).

Obviously, one drawback with this type of exercise is expense—you need access to a club or to buy the machine yourself to put it in your home. I'd recommend both (the club first to get acclimated, then purchase the machine after you are satisfied, and keep the membership).

It will be the best investment you ever made (along with the reclined exercise bicycle!). Several thousand dollars for machines is only a tenth of the cost of a good car these days, should last longer, and will pay health dividends far beyond the initial cost.

The results will appreciate and not *depreciate* like a new car!

I've watched people in the gym—even people who look like they'd know better—waste hours jerking weights around, slamming them, using too little weight to do any good, too much, and just wasting their time (it doesn't do the weights or my hearing any good either!).

So, we've already covered a method to burn calories safely and efficiently to get the results we need. We have a method to increase our strength and work capacity safely, practically, and efficiently, and repetitive *work is what burns calories.*

We have come a long way along one half of the "calories in, calories out" equation. Before we get to the other half—food—let's reinforce one of the main concepts in this book. Then, we'll explore some mental issues that may be barriers to our success.

Take home points:

Progressive resistive exercises—to build strength—enhance work capacity, aerobic conditioning, and thus calorie burning.

The fifteen repetitions maximum, done correctly, will offer intensity without getting bored, and results.

You must feel the burn, and progressively increase your weight over the ensuing weeks and months. You must do the exercises SLOWLY.

SLOWLY . . . SLOWLY . . . SLOWLY . . .

Chapter 4: Intensity is Key

All you out there—no matter how old or what your background is—need to work out (aerobic and strength training) in one way: WITH SUFFICIENT *INTENSITY*.

I've given you all kinds of cues as to when you are working intensively. You should consult your doctor and your trainer—but you have a good idea of when that is.

But, to be honest, for most, it's when you start to feel *out of your comfort zone* (I'm not talking chest pain here—you've consulted your doctor already!)

You don't like feeling *uncomfortable*. None of us do (actually, not true—but that is a tangent). For most, even a "gentle burn" is to be avoided.

However, I propose to you, and please trust the process (you have to trust *something*, don't you? besides, what have you got to loose, really?) that as you loose weight and gain strength and your body acclimates to the intense work, you *will stop* feeling uncomfortable.

You will *like* the burn!

Your discomfort will turn into something else: satisfaction, even exhilaration!

Some call it a warm buzz—some call it a pleasant burn—like scratching something hard that itches. Some call it like an org . . . never mind, you got the idea!

I know, some of the ladies out there are shaking their heads and quipping that this is only a "male" or testosterone thing: right? Not true.

Millions of years of evolution and killing the sloths for the cave dinner; Venus and Mars; and male masochism psychobabble . . . rubbish! It doesn't matter if you're a man or woman or a hermaphrodite. The pleasure of the pleasant burn shall be with you, especially when your endorphins start kicking in.

It may help if, when you start out on your program, you don't think of training as a hobby, but as an adventuresome battle (yes, women too!).

Hobbies are really things like painting, sailing, writing (unless you sell something—then it's a vocation), martial arts, knitting, and the like—things we should be doing in good health to distract us from life's warts.

However, battles can be pleasurable too (they must be: read a history book or a newspaper)—it's in our DNA. The key is to redirect this aggressive energy to your fat, and not yourself or others. The old, "calories in, calories out" battle—far older than the invention of the refrigerator itself—is part of fitness.

Fitness (I submit) is a no-nonsense business—*life's business*—and not a hobby (at least until you get your first twenty-five to thirty pounds off with increased strength, stamina, and less disease). Then, you can make it a hobby.

Ideally, once you've gotten tucked into your program—let's say—by using your favorite club, and you like it, invest some money in good home machines. You know what those are.

Find a quiet corner of your house at any convenient time: lock the door; put on the headphones and your favorite music; and—three to six times per week—go through your aerobic and weight training program. To be more focused, forget the headphones.

The whole thing should take just under an hour, including gentle stretches. Concentrate on your specific muscles and your body *every second* of that allotted time. Pump the weights, burn the butt, breathe evenly and deeply.

Try to enjoy the *intense* work until you feel the soft burn and the endorphins kick in. With proper diet, in three to six months your body will start to transform into something different—something better.

You'll become addicted to this—better this than Almond Joys or cocaine.

Take home points:

Work out intensively in less time. Consider wearing earplugs instead of headphones in the gym to facilitate focus. Wal-Mart has great ones.

Without intensity, you are largely wasting your valuable time and money.

Work out intensively.

Work out intensively.

Work out intensively.

Work out . . . well, you've got the idea.

Chapter 5: Depression and Addiction

We must talk about this, because for many it gets in the way of results. Most of the chapters in this book incorporate some issues of attitude and philosophy—and are to some degree subjective. This one is especially so. Some of this dabbling can be useful. Why? Attitude can defeat our plan.

For serious cases of depression and addiction, you must consult the proper health care professionals, such as physicians, psychologists, and others. Depression is a major killer (suicide), and must be addressed pronto by experts in that field.

Sometimes there's a thin line between depression, addiction, and extreme moods, all of which may interfere with our enjoyment of life. Moreover, does addiction cause depression, or the other way around, or both? When are moods excessive and dangerous? What is the best prevention for many kinds of depression or addiction? What treatments work best?

You must consult your board certified psychiatrist or psychologist for the best answers to these questions.

However, at the margin, for most of us, simple, safe, and practical ways to live our lives can help navigate us away from some of these common mental afflictions—or assist in controlling them.

I would contend that proper exercise, diet, and sound sleep hygiene (which is impacted by both and impacts both), form the kernel of these ways.

We must remember that it's very hard to prove this from a scientific standpoint.

This is due to the fact that medical studies are very difficult and expensive to design—especially for this subjective topic. There are too many variables to control. How do we measure these things reliably? However, intuition, experience, and anecdotal evidence from our *own* lives can often be instructive.

Eliminating for the time being the dietary side of the equation, intense exercise—aerobic and strengthening—may be effective in lessening the impact of addictive and depressive impulses.

First, you must be aware of these impulses, and the bits of behavior in which they manifest.

Downing one martini after another, buying the big bag of candy bars at Costco, taking more pain pills than prescribed, you must focus on what you are *doing* that is harmful. You must be *aware*. The topic of "Mindfulness" will be discussed briefly in a later chapter—but it essentially says: "live your day in the *present and be aware*."

Generally, they say that depression is chemical or situational, or both. It's probable that intense exercise can positively impact all types. What unhealthy mental impulses trigger these malfunctions in our mental capacity?

Is it internalized anger, or internalized aggression, or aggression that has no channel of expression, or lack of healthy sleep, or memories of a bad childhood, or all the above, or what?

Whatever it is exactly, it's likely that its effects on functioning—the final common pathway—can be impacted by intense exercise. It is probable that proper diet magnifies or facilitates these positive effects.

Can I prove it *statistically* and *scientifically* beyond a shadow of a doubt? Probably not, but I don't need to, because it works.

We sense that addiction and depression are close cousins from a causation standpoint, but just how? Well, that is way beyond the scope of this book, and I don't have a clue anyway. But, we can sidestep those answers by remembering that the bottom-line is how we *feel* and *function*.

Again, I believe that intense exercise can positively impact how we feel and function in the grips of either disorder.

This may be great news, since one very destructive form of addiction is *overeating*. Furthermore, overeating can depress any of us.

It is likely that as you progress with this program, and loose weight, gain strength, and improve your diet and your appearance, your impulses to "overeat" will diminish—therefore hastening your results. You will feel more upbeat. You probably will feel less "depressed."

However, if you are under a psychiatrist's care, their advice overrides anything in the book—so listen.

The best way to unleash the positive power of intense exercise is to perform them early in the morning, so we feel the pleasant burn of our muscles and experience the endorphin highs much of the day. This helps us to ward off those destructive impulses facilitating depression and addiction. Its metabolism stimulating properties also allows us to passively burn more calories throughout the day.

This takes time—so do not expect results overnight. Give yourself six months.

Besides food, there are other, more life-threatening addictions of course, such as alcohol, street drugs, non-street drugs, and the like, all beyond the scope of this book. Probably, these disorders can be helped with intense exercise and proper diet, along with other treatments. Lessening these addictions can aid our program results.

You must consult the proper health care professionals

The more senses you engage in a positive way while exercising, the more the intensity of your workouts may ward off the "evil spirits" of depression and addiction. Try arranging the colors and shapes of your exercise room in vibrant, complementary colors, with decorations that have uplifting shapes, tones, and textures.

Don't forget your favorite picture of your healthy mascot: the orangutan!

Why not hang copies of impressionist paintings? Why not burn your favorite incense or arrange your favorite scented flowers too (come on guys, you love it!)?

Why not wear cashmere gloves or underwear while you do your exercises? Well, perhaps . . .

Last, the issue of healthy sleep is important.

Unhealthy or inadequate sleep—perhaps deranged in some ways that we don't yet fully understand—likely contributes not only to addiction and depression but other *physical* diseases as well. (*sleep, deprivation, disorders, medical, depression, addiction, etiology, cause, studies, articles*).

One such important and common *physical* disease we will visit later in this book (see Chapter 8). It's vital to your exercise program, and to your general health, that you reserve enough time for adequate and restful sleep under the best conditions possible.

Patients with depression and addiction must be cleared for intense exercise too. After all, being depressed doesn't protect you from a heart attack.

Take home points:

Depression and addiction, especially in its moderate forms, may respond to intensive exercise—especially aerobic exercise.

Be aware of what bad behaviors generate addictive and depressive impulses, and vice versa.

Addiction and depression may be closely linked.

Consider discussing with your analyst, if you have one, some of the topics discussed in this chapter.

Chapter 6: Orangutan Diet

Well, here we are: calories *in*: food.

Weight *loss* is the key to your health, and, for most of us, the key to this is diet. So, this is probably one of the most important chapters in this book. It's vital to get your hands around this issue as you progress with other things, not *after*.

Most "experts" will tell you that the best exercise to loose weight is to push yourself away from the dinner table—and there's some truth in that.

But, there are effective and ineffective ways to do it. You will *not* go hungry.

The trick is to form new habits that are good, and discard ones which are bad—without hunger.

Read on.

Yes, I know, you are really healthy, you never get a cold, and you look thick in the middle but basically "good" for fifty.

However, your doctor tells you that you are overweight, have high blood pressure, and your labs are marginal at best.

You *must* loose weight, she insists. But you protest. You're *only* 230 pounds—after all—and you're *almost* six foot tall and *muscular*, right? You've *only* gained twenty pounds since you played ball in college. You work out with weights and jog a little too.

Who needs to loose weight?
You do.

The women reading this book have their own version of this story.

I don't care what is muscle and what is not, how you *think* you look (not really as good as you suppose), how few colds you catch, or how far you "jog"—you need to lose *pounds*—any pounds at first.

That's it!

Unless you play linebacker for the Cleveland Browns, the loss also needs to be a lot more than ten pounds. You and your doctor must decide, but you need to get down, in this example, to 200 or so at least—for now.

I know, you've tried small portions, fasting, swimming, the fruit plan, the liquid diet plan, on and on and it doesn't work. Actually, you did loose a lot of weight once, but you gained it all back pronto and then some.

Well, trust *this* plan—trust the process, give it a chance, give it three months—not three weeks. After all, you've got to put your faith in something, right? Why not this?

Now I'd like to introduce you to two important concepts: the *Giant, Orangutan Vegetable Stewpot*: and the *Giant Orangutan Wok.* They're not overly original, not fancy, not esoteric, but are safe, inexpensive, time-efficient, simple—and most importantly—they will *work*.

This method will also control your sodium intake and doesn't require learning a bunch of new recipes, calculating, measuring, recording, hours of tending, and a slew of extra dirty dishes to clean.

If you must binge at first, you can do it with them, not cheesecake!

I can just hear the guffaws and chuckles out there. These items are not exactly out of one of those fancy fitness magazines or expensive health club newsletters. Don't knock it until you've tried it—and for three months at least!

It is lasting results you want, not art.

Now, let's get to some details.

Orangutans, while burning their butts and other large muscle groups while climbing around in trees and over hill and dale, consume large quantities of vegetation. This includes fruits, nuts, herbs, veggies, bark, twigs, and apparently the odd insect or bird egg or Big Mac (so they are not *strictly* herbivores).

Go to Costco (or equivalent store) and buy the *huge* cooking pot—the stainless steel one with the copper inlay for good heat distribution.

If they have a similar huge wok, buy that too. If not, go to your favorite Asian store and buy one. Do *not* buy a pot or a wok with plastic coating on the inside. Make sure they both come with covers.

Next, go to the vegetable section of Costco (or your favorite store) and buy the following ingredients: one large package each of fresh (refrigerated) raw, precut broccoli; carrots; cauliflower; Brussels sprouts; dark mushrooms; green beans; multi-colored peppers; and chard, spinach, or cabbage (or all three if you like). Grab a big bag of onions and a clump of garlic (if bad breath is no issue).

Add or substitute your favorite fresh (never frozen) vegetables that you see in the large cooler section.

Next, go to the fruit section. Buy a large package of apples, plums, pears, or grapes. I like these because they're portioned and easy to eat without making a mess or having to clean a dish.

Remember, life is easy!

Next, go to the soup section and buy a pack of vegetable soup (if you are a vegetarian, *vegetarian* vegetable soup) to go into the vegetable stew as a base stock. Near that section of the store, you'll see the canned beans somewhere (grab a clerk to help you).

Now we add the proteins.

Ordinarily, I'm against canned anything, but there are exceptions. Canned vegetables have a large amount of sodium in them, and if they have a lower sodium version, use that. At Costco, buy a large pack of Rosarita canned, vegetarian refried beans (buy the vegetarian version even if you are not a vegetarian— it's lower in fat and cholesterol). This is an excellent source of fiber and protein and will go into your strew stock for added flavor and body.

Get over to the refrigerated tofu section and buy a block of non-fried tofu—firm curd. If you see cans of garbanzo and kidney beans packed in water, get those—otherwise obtain them at your favorite grocery store.

Those sources of fiber and protein go into your stew—after you drained them of the water from the can (or light sauce—not packed in oil!). You can cook dried beans but that takes time so forget it. Get a bag of your favorite *brown* or *wild* rice (non-white rice is usually higher in fiber, protein, and flavor).

Ordinarily, starches will play little role in our weight control program and diet, but this is an exception.

Brown or wild rice, and cornstarch, are nice choices to thicken the vegetable stew and give it body, flavor, texture, and added nutrients. Brown rice—each portion of which should be no larger than your fist when cooked—is a nice adjunct to your prepared wok dinners.

In weight control, starches, such as potatoes, are even bigger offenders than fats like butter, cheese, milk, egg yolks, cream cheese, creams, and the like. It seems there's a natural limit to the volume of fats most of us can consume—even for the most glutinous.

The same is *not* true of starches.

The feedbag is endless when it comes to starches like spaghetti, any potato, fresh breads, roles, and even rice (so be careful!).

This does not even mention most *sweet* bakery goods, where starches, sugars, *and* fats abound.

Starches are the kiss of death to any successful weight control plan, and they are much stealthier than good old steaks or cheesecake. I've seen many dieters shovel a quart of mashed potatoes onto their plate and call it healthy, just because they didn't use butter with it!

In contrast, not many of us would call a slice of cheesecake "healthy."

Personally, I've never met a potato I didn't like—taboo for you (at least for now)!

Now, go to the meat section and buy low sodium turkey (or chicken) *real* breast—already sliced. Costco has a brand of sliced turkey that may be highly suitable. If you are a vegetarian, obviously skip this step. You may dice these into small portions and get them ready for the stewpot (or wok).

I will now list other miscellaneous, sundry ingredients and materials that are recommended for your use. You may purchase these at Costco or any good grocery store. I would also strongly consider a good Asian or international grocery store for a wider variety of exotic veggies, herbs, and spices.

The ingredients and materials are (we shall get to the assembly and cooking presently): large wooden and metal spoons without plastic coatings; large, sharp carving and chopping knives; a large wooden carving board; and a big, metal soup ladle. You also need olive or peanut oil (both can cook at very high temperatures); *fresh* cilantro, mint, basil, rosemary, and oregano herbs, paprika, cinnamon, nutmeg, chipotle, cayenne pepper, and chili powder spices.

Red, yellow, and green curry paste and powder (try them all), cans of light coconut milk, and a small jar of Skippy Extra Chunky peanut butter (hands off—just for the pot!) is also recommended. Fresh limes and lemons and coarsely ground black pepper, fresh, grated Parmesan and Romano cheese, and Laughing Cow light, creamy Swiss cheese triangles (each is a portion) are useful as well.

What's this about cheese, you ask? Well, in small, low fat amounts, traces of select cheese can add a lot of flavor, body, and satisfaction with little adverse impact. Think of it as a culinary vaccine!

I would also stock Heinz steak sauce, Heinz 57 and Heinz Chili sauces, spicy mustard with horseradish, and Worcestershire (have you ever tried to spell that word!) sauce all for the Yankee version of the vegetable stewpot. To this you can add a dash of grated cheese or a cheese triangle for the pot seasoning. If you have favorite seasonings, try them.

I recommend any or all of the following flavorings—*minus* as much sodium and MSG as you can find. These flavorings are (and you can substitute them with your favorites): vegetarian Hoisin sauce; chili soy paste; Sriracha and sweet chili sauce; light soy sauce (low sodium); Bangkok peanut sauce; and soy bean sauce and paste.

Usually, vegetarian versions of these sauces have less fat and less mystery meats.

The basic principle behind the vegetable stew pot is to use herbs, spices, flavorings, and sauces that are pungent, spicy (if you like that—I do), and satisfying, so that your large vegetable stew portion is appetizing and SATISFYING.

These flavors carry a big punch.

These ingredients, remember, are going to be diluted into huge volumes, so even though some of them are not particularly low sodium or low fat choices, when massively diluted—they're acceptable. The vegetable stew will have little of the concentrated sodium, fat, and calorie content that you see in canned or highly processed foods.

It's important that you experiment and find the right flavor combinations for you—there are no rules here.

The wok has similar principles.

However, "solid" food—as from a wok—tends to satisfy us more than less solid food, so the wok meal is saved for the evening meal. The stewpot will be used for breakfast and lunch and snacks, and the wok vegetables and rice will be consumed later—around seven o'clock or so.

Some, however, will prefer to have their "solid" meal during lunch, and not in the evening. That's fine.

For those of you who cannot stomach a huge portion of seasoned vegetables early in the morning, you may substitute four hard-boiled eggs, without salt, removing three and a half yolks before you eat them all. You may distribute the half yolk between all the solid egg white, to get some in each bite. These egg whites may also be consumed as snacks—for good protein and some essential fat content.

I recommend eating at seven in the evening for the "main" meal, and not earlier, because we don't want to wake up hungry.

There are no snacks after the evening meal, except for one or two pieces of fruit. Ten minutes before your fruit, drink one large glass of filtered water.

In fact, it's essential that you drink as much *water* during the day as possible—preferably a few minutes *before* you eat and not after. This blunts the ravenous appetite, and won't interfere with the natural digestive juices. Do you ever see orangutans (or any other animal) drinking anything while they eat? Even animals that catch their prey by rivers and streams don't seem to do that.

Buy a very large Thermos and load it with your hot vegetable stew each day, and take it with you to work or where ever you are during lunchtime. Do not go hungry! Eat a huge portion.

Why not? It's mostly green vegetables and water and satisfying seasonings. Eat as much vegetable stew as you like, but eat it *slowly*!

I recommend buying a cake timer, and forcing yourself to eat all your meals in *not faster than thirty minutes*! Concentrate on each bite, with minimal distractions—including no *loud* music or phones present! Turn off the boob tube and computer screens.

"Mindfulness" suggests: concentrate on each second of eating like treasure that will never return (actually it *will* never—and it *is*).

Mindfulness suggests that we only really live in a series of moments in the *present*—not the past or the future (*Mindfulness, philosophy, psychology, tenets, beliefs, proponents, addiction, food, practical use, anxiety*). How can your food be satisfying if your mind is in the future or the past all the time?

If you're not satisfied, you'll stuff more calories down your gullet. That makes it difficult to loose weight and to keep it off.

Fruit can be very misleading. Fruit should be treated as a treat—and a desert. Many people think that natural fruit is almost calorie free and very healthy. The truth is, the sugar calories from fruit can add up fast to diet-busting proportions—especially fruit *juices*.

I know—the sugar is *natural* you say, so it's ok. No, it is not ok! A huge glass of fresh-squeezed orange juice has a whopping amount of calories, and you only get so many calories during the day! (*juices, calories, fruit, portions*). Be sensible and consider your fruit intake as being "nature's desert."

Nuts are another source of fantasy. They are natural and healthy, right? Eat all you want. Wrong—the calories can add up fast, so if you use them for the pot, crush a few up and use caution.

So, what do we do with these ingredients and materials?

Take them home; put your big pot on the kitchen counter after you filled it with water half way. Take your packages of precut vegetables, put them in a strainer and run water over them, drain them, and dump each vegetable in the pot. Do not cut them any more before you do this.

Dump one can of Rosarita refried beans into the pot, with one can of vegetable soup, one cup of brown rice, a can of coconut milk lite, and a dollop of cornstarch and peanut oil. Dump in a can of strained garbanzo beans too. Put in one large spoonful of peanut butter and two or three dollops of curry paste. If you detest any of these ingredients, use something else.

There are no taste rules here.

Put in finely chopped, fresh basil, onion, cilantro, and garlic (if breath is not an issue).

Now, fill the rest of the pot with water—almost to the top. Take your hot sauce and squirt it in to taste, along with any or all the Asian seasonings and spices you like. There are no rules—*the rule is that your taste buds like it!*

I love to finely chop and mince a juicy slice of lime—with the peel and pulp—then throw it in. It tastes simply divine!

If you're a compulsive personality, and must measure and dirty every utensil in the kitchen to feel whole, you can do so. Your cleanup will be longer, but go ahead.

It's unnecessary.

Just get it done and gain experience while you experiment. It'll be more fun without the fuss and won't drain your energy. Now, turn the fire under the pot on medium for about twenty minutes (in the mean time, do something relaxing)—until it boils—then stir the pot thoroughly.

At this stage, you can take your sharp knife and slice the vegetables *in the pot* to a thinner consistency if you like, without dirtying dishes.

Just trap the veggies against the side of the pot with your knife, and pretend it's the cable guy (just kidding!). Actually, this step may be unnecessary, since the vegetables largely break up eventually. That is up to your taste buds.

After that, lower the flame to simmer for about two hours (with the cover open a crack to let the aroma out). Go do your exercises, read your book, or attend to your hobby! When you return, you'll have a huge pot of vegetable stew done and ready to go—and for half of the week!

Grab a *big* bowl and consume a *huge* portion—*slowly*—in not less than thirty minutes. Think about *every* bite!

If you don't like Asian flavors (you probably will acquire a taste for it however—Thai is my favorite), try an Italian theme. If you don't like that, then eat Mexican. If not that, then try good old Yankee flavors. If not that . . . well, you got the idea.

If you like all of them switch every couple of days. You have the main ingredients in your cupboard and refrigerator. Some get to like just the vegetables without any seasoning—just natural—except maybe a low fat, low salt cracker, or two. Some like heavy variations of mustard (which has few calories)!

You should consume all the stew within three days. If necessary, discard what's left and do it over again to maintain freshness. By the way, you are saving a ton of money on your grocery bill.

Preparing the meal with the huge wok is similar. Take the wok and put it under a maximal flame after squirting in a small dollop of peanut oil.

When that is very hot (after a few minutes), throw in a dash of curry paste, garlic, and chili paste. Let the whole thing liquefy, and then throw in the veggies in the same manner as the stew, plus any extra seasonings, flavorings, and spices. The flame must be kept at maximal, rapidly stirring the veggies with your favorite spoon.

Do *not* add water!

Cover the mixture for about five minutes to let the veggies soften. Take off the cover, this time adding finely chopped basil, cilantro, curry powder, coconut milk lite, and a little chunky peanut butter. Take your sharp knife and cut the veggies against the wall of the wok—just as you did for the stewpot.

This is why you don't want a plastic coated pot or wok—it may come off right into your food with stirring or cutting! Besides, if you submerge your pot and wok in water right after you cook (if you don't use it as a storage container—which I do), and you used a small, negligible amount of oil to minimize sticking, both should be easy to clean.

Wok the whole thing for another five to ten minutes or so, and you are done! You now have a huge wok full of food that lasts for half the week!

Now, five minutes before you started cooking with your wok, you should have taken two or three cups (I don't need a *measuring* cup) of brown rice and dump it into a small pot. You immerse the rice so that the waterline is just slightly over the layer of dry rice. Put the pot on a high flame until it boils.

Then, you cover and simmer it on a low flame for about thirty minutes or so—until the rice is tender and your wok food is done. No messing, no measuring, and no fussing—just do it.

Now, since your wok food is done, and your rice is done, take a big plate, put a fist-size portion of rice on it, and smother it with the wonderful wok vegetables—a *huge* portion. For gluttons, you may have a portion of *pot* vegetables *before* your meal—to appease your appetite. Why not?

Drink a large glass of water as you set the table before you eat. Enjoy the food with no distractions. Think about each tasty morsel. You may ponder how you might improve it the next time, or maybe use a different theme—such as Italian or Mexican style vegetables.

If the wok and pot are huge enough, and it should be, you'll have all your breakfast, lunch (remember the big Thermos), and dinner for the next three days—plus extra portions during the day if you get hungry. As you use up your vegetable pot, dilute the rest with water until the three days are up—so it's more like a soup. This will make it last, and each portion will have slightly less calories and sodium.

In this diet, the key is *a large portion*—not a small one. You will never go hungry!

Anyone in the restaurant business knows that if a customer leaves hungry she will never come back.

The same is true in dieting. Leave the table hungry too many times, and you'll never return to the weight control plan. We don't want that.

We didn't say much about meat. How about the turkey, chicken, or even tofu—which isn't meat? Well, put it in if you like, and be sparing with the tofu. Too much isn't good for men—and it does have significant calories. If you like tofu, chop it into small squares and put a little in your wok or stewpot.

Cut the turkey and chicken slices into little strips or cubes, and put them in too if you like. Although there is already protein in the ingredients, extra protein—particularly animal protein—can be desirable in the right form such as this.

There are no taste rules, just what you like!

The wok, the Thermos, the stewpot, the fruit, the water, the cooked egg whites, and coffee in the morning if you drink it, will be the source of your food for the next six months—until you loose the twenty-five to thirty pounds.

You'll find that your taste buds will change, and so will your cravings. The vegetables, in time, will seem more satisfying and substantial—and wholesome. You'll feel good after you eat, not just during. You'll look forward to your big wok and pot meals more and more.

After all, orangutans never ate hamburgers and fries (most didn't anyway!).

You don't need them either.

Don't cheat—stick to the program—you'll not be disappointed. After all (you know the mantra by now), you have to believe in something, don't you? Put your trust in it and it will reward you.

This isn't flashy, but it works. It is results that you are after, not art (you've heard this jingle too!).

At a minimum, promise yourself that you'll give it a three-month, earnest trial. You'll be happy you did. Remember replacing bad habits with good? Your new habits are the wok and vegetable pot.

After you take off the initial thirty pounds or so, then you can decide to continue to the next thirty—and I hope you do.

You must ask yourself at that time just how you'll keep the weight off if you do *not* go on with this plan? I hope you will conclude that the best way is to incorporate our plan into your life for good, and not just for the next thirty pounds (if you and your doctor agree).

Moreover, at the six-month mark (if you go on to the next thirty pounds or just want to maintain what you have using this plan), you'll have the option of one "free" day per week, and one "free meal" per day—within reason. During these days, you can eat almost anything you like, in moderate portions.

However, to balance the calories, you'll probably have to increase the intensity of your aerobic workouts a bit, and the duration (or modify your recipes—read on). Out-of-town vacations (and major holidays) are the same—up to two weeks per year—free time within reason.

When that time comes though, I bet most of you will *not* take total advantage of those days that are "free." You'll have changed your habits and acclimated to the new signals that you are getting from your improved body (and taste buds).

You will also be delighted with the medical "fringe benefits" that will accrue to the new you (chapters 8 and 10).

But, until then, you have work to do.

Take home lessons:

The key is *big* portions, and not small ones.

Eat an appetizer of a pot portion before you start your evening wok meal if you like. Don't eat too early.

Use one or two pieces of fruit as desert or treats an hour or so before bedtime.

Pack your *big* lunch portion of vegetable stew.

Make sure all your portions are hot! Hot food is inherently more satisfying. Drink a large glass of cold water ten minutes *before* eating, and eat slowly.

Give this *at least* a three-month trial—you'll need six months with this whole program for thirty pounds.

As your condition changes, so will your taste buds. Never load your refrigerator with such things as breads, cakes, pies, mashed potatoes, or steaks (at least for six months anyway).

An inexpensive multi-vitamin from Wal-Mart won't hurt, with trace minerals and any supplement that your doctor orders (example: calcium for ladies with osteoporosis).

Chapter 7: Goals; Chemicals; Sodium

Remember, the goal is to loose weight and with it bulk. Food can be considered the biggest drug around, and it can have adverse effects just as prescription medications do. I don't just mean putting on fat. Sodium and chemicals are some of processed food's potentially harmful side effects.

Almost all processed food is loaded with sodium. It's a true pandemic. Even low fat, low calorie choices in upscale grocery and "health food" stores are often packed with even more sodium to "enhance" flavor. Shoppers might suspect: " . . . if we can't load customers with calories, we'll make up for it with salt!"

Go to the chips section (on one of your "free days") of your favorite grocery store, and see how many choices they have for low fat, low calorie, *and* low sodium chips. You'll find one if you're lucky. The same is true of popcorn.

Packing sodium into our foods is a major contributor to high blood pressure. High blood pressure is rampant, especially in the over forty crowd. High blood pressure puts you at greater risk for kidney disease, heart disease, and strokes.

The good news is that your vegetable stewpot and wok food are very low in sodium, even if you have a few higher sodium flavorings mixed in the broth—due to the *huge* dilution effects.

However, you should always try to use low sodium versions of seasonings and sauces, or lower sodium substitutes. It's true that some vegetables are higher in sodium content (*sodium, content, high, vegetables, whole, unprocessed, raw, FDA*), but it shrinks in importance compared to processed foods. Also, we have the higher sodium veggies diluted with the lower content ones.

It's usually obvious which are the high sodium foods in the grocery store, and we must avoid them (you will anyway with orangutan weight control). Read the labels. Chips, pickles, most canned foods, soups, most sauces, jarred veggies, almost any processed meat product, and prepared dinners (frozen or not) typically have tons of sodium.

Sodium is a killer so observe your limits. Daily requirements of sodium are: (*sodium, food content, FDA recommendations, daily, allowance*). Fresh lemon squeezed onto your food is often a tasty, healthy salt substitute. Try it.

Chemicals are maybe even harder to eliminate from the grocery products we buy at the store, and unfortunately, we may not even know what chemicals are really in them. This includes both product additives deliberately put in the food, and chemicals that may be sprayed on the food at different stages of its production (pesticides, fertilizers, and "freshening" treatments).

We can try to buy "organic" vegetables from reputable stores, but do the stores really know exactly what "organic" means? Do we?

Does "organic" really mean with *no* pesticides? I ask my grocer these questions and it doesn't seem like anyone is sure. We pay for the organic label, but are we really getting it?

Who enforces the rules, even if we know what organic means? You believe what you want, but I'm not sure that is happening. The bottom line is you must thoroughly wash all vegetables before they go in the pot or wok.

You must read the label carefully of the foods you buy. Sometimes it's hard to compare because portion sizes and weight systems may be non-standardized, so take your calculator and conversion table to the store with you.

So what? Can these chemicals in the food harm us?

The answer is that probably we don't know—but it's wise to error on the side of caution.

It's hard to design valid studies that test whether these contaminants (or ingredients such as non-nutritive sweeteners and synthetic food colorings) are harmful or not in the long run (aside from taste issues). It takes years (and big dollars) and thousands of test subjects—with strictly controlled variables—to even come close to obtaining valid data.

In the meantime, error on the side of caution and eliminate them the best you can (unless your doctor prescribes such foods, for diabetics, let's say).

Also, watch what you are putting on your skin. Try to use natural products. The human skin is a very large source of drug (and contaminant) absorption. Many lotions and creams are packed with chemicals and high-energy compounds that, theoretically, are perhaps fertile ground to contribute to cancer risk.

The cheap (and varied) plastics used in today's packaging of food products or in saving portions at home are another potential source of concern. Personally, I never heat up anything in plastic, either in the oven or microwave. I don't care what the instructions say. Heat your food using conventional dishes.

Liquid packaged in plastic cartons, like milk, often has shavings that come off in your milk when you unscrew the cap, so beware.

Orangutans (in the wild anyway) don't use bad lotions or eat farm grown veggies with harmful pesticides, so you shouldn't either.

Take home lessons:

Thoroughly wash all your veggies before eating them.

Buy your "organic" veggies at the highest quality "health food" or grocery store you can. Many mainline grocery stores, like Ralphs, have "healthy" offerings. Wholefoods is a wonderful place, and it, like Ralphs, has the market power to control quality.

Be cautious about what you put on your skin—some potentially suspect compounds can be absorbed into your bloodstream.

Eliminating sodium from your diet is extremely difficult. One of the best ways to do this is with the Orangutan wok and veggie stewpot.

Beware of non-nutritive sweeteners. I have no evidence of direct harm, but again, why not error on the side of caution? For example, if you need a good soda without calories, try the brands with the natural sweetener from the stevia plant. These are more expensive, but it's only money, right? Well . . .

Chapter 8: Killers: Sleep Apnea; HTN

Sleep apnea and HTN (hypertension—high blood pressure) are very common medical disorders that usually go hand in hand. Both are highly correlated with being overweight, and both can be deadly over time. A thirty-pound excess is enough to be a major risk factor for sleep apnea, which commonly presents in middle age or after.

Sleep apnea is a condition whereby the airway of the person usually closes while asleep, leading to restriction of oxygen to the brain and abrupt awakening. This leads to seriously disordered sleep and often presents with a slew of other hazardous medical disorders, such as impaired mental functioning, hypertension, accelerated coronary artery disease (potential for heart attacks), and a significantly increased risk for stroke.

Sleep apnea is probably far more common than supposed, and the patient will display loud snoring, jerking while asleep, choking sounds, and severe insomnia with irritability.

Stroke and heart attacks, with cancer, are major causes of death, especially in the over forty crowd.

So, sleep apnea is a killer, and the best, direct treatment for it is—in most of the population—significant weight loss. For mild to moderate cases of sleep apnea, a thirty-pound weight loss could be curative. Other, more invasive treatments are surgery and bedside breathing equipment. Drugs, with potentially unpleasant side effects, are also used to combat the insomnia secondary to sleep apnea.

As far as stroke is concerned, the risk factors are well defined, and most of them are highly correlated with being overweight.

These are: high blood pressure; high cholesterol; diabetes; smoking; atrial fibrillation; excessively fat diet; lack of exercise; and family history. Key labs, which reflect these risk factors, and which should be monitored by your doctor are: Total Cholesterol; HDL Cholesterol; LDL Cholesterol; Blood Glucose levels; Triglycerides; and others. Other conditions that correlate with increased risk for stoke are abdominal aortic aneurysm and carotid artery occlusion, which can be monitored using non-invasive ultrasound and physical exam.

Fats, excessive salt, sedentary lifestyle, alcohol, may all contribute to hypertension, diabetes, and stroke risk, as well as to the major killer: coronary artery disease. In fact, obesity is being correlated more and more with an increased risk for some cancers, yet more killers—need I go on?

Folks, it's time to loose the thirty pounds. It's time to ensure a higher quality of sleep and to prevent or treat sleep apnea.

It's time to get started on the Orangutan Weight Control program!

While we are on the subject of sleep, we need to recognize the importance of sleep hygiene in general with regard to our ability to progress with the plan. Restful, nourishing, restorative sleep is one of the vital underpinnings of emotional wellbeing and properly functioning mental and physical capacity—including exercise.

It's difficult to prove, but sound sleep—and enough of it—is essential to thwart disease and prevent mental illness.

Stress, anxiety, depression, addictive behaviors, stimulants, alcohol, smoking, drugs, and bad habits all contribute to sleep disturbance. If you find yourself unable to secure enough quality sleep for whatever reason—with or without sleep apnea—you need to consult a top sleep center in your community.

Often, medical directors of these centers are Board Certified Pulmonologists or Neurologists. They will perform a complete history and physical, medical record review, and probably order an overnight "sleep study," before recommending treatment. Your primary care doctor can refer you to such a center.

It's important that you get the right professional help. Sleep is one of the few things that you can't "will yourself" to do. In fact, the harder one tries to sleep, the more it evades you.

Take home lessons:

Sleep apnea—and the diseases associated with it including hypertension—is a dangerous condition. Thirty pounds of weight loss for many can the most effective and safe treatment.

Chapter 9: Stress, Anxiety, "Mindfulness"

Is there any doubt that a lot of overeating is due to stress and anxiety? It is also getting clearer in medicine that the stress and anxiety of modern living is impacting our basic physiology in terms of hormonal levels and metabolic functioning, not to mention general health and disease states.

Again, this is hard to prove. We are getting into voodoo. Also, how do we measure stress? How do you control the variables that apply to stress? How do you measure tiny physiologic responses to subtle changes in anxiety states—*reliably*?

Forget about the cost, the design of such studies is devilishly hard.

Yet, I'm as sure about the fact that these things impact our ability to live healthy lives as I am about the sun coming up tomorrow. The question is: *how* do we control stress and anxiety?

I love it when doctors tell us to eliminate our stress. They know we can't. What they mean of course is to develop strategies to manage it.

I see stress and anxiety as two sides of the same coin. I see much of anxiety as stress that we can't manage, and so we fret about it. It's also fear of the unknown—things we can't control—that overwhelm us.

So, how do we manage these things? How do we get more control? The answer to this is extremely personal and individualized, and I'll leave it to you to figure out the details. However, a few generalizations may be helpful.

First, recognize that stress and anxiety is a big health problem. Be aware of what you are doing and how you are thinking and feeling at any given *moment* when you feel stressed and anxious. Are there things in the present around you that are bothering you *now*?

Second, realize that most of our fretting, anxiety, and feeling of helplessness is not triggered by events happening *now* (PRESENT tense), but rather dwelling upon stressful things that *have happened* to us (PAST tense) or *will* happen to us (FUTURE tense). In other words, we are consumed with tomorrow and the anticipation of stress or lack of control, which is itself stressful and makes us anxious. Alternatively, we may be anxious about the stressful things that happened last week.

But right *now*—are we ok? Are we bankrupt, bleeding, or dying? If not, why *not* enjoy every second of the present, and not be consumed with the past and future?

The answer of course to all of this is to learn to be more focused on the PRESENT, like orangutans do. I've never met a neurotic orangutan. Why? They only think in the present tense (I suppose—I can't really prove it). Take a bite out of that bark, swallow that bug, and swing on the branch to hide! That's it, not: *will I have the money to buy bananas next year?*

It seems that this is what much of the present "mindfulness" movement is generally about—at least to me. In various forms, similar philosophies have surfaced for decades. This one is packaged differently, but still holds. I think there's a lot to be said for it. So, how do we implement this?

That's for you to study and figure out for yourself (try: *mindfulness, psychology, application, process, implementation, anxiety, uses*). One thought: intense exercise forces us to think in the present!

If we are trying to remove things that we can't control, why not remove much of the "media"? Not all of it of course (like this book or TCN or HBO!), but just those parts of it that are consumed with negative energy, unsubstantiated "truth", and violent emotions that plunge us into the dark future and the murky past—thus adding to our anxiety and stress.

This is not to say that you should be an ostrich. An ostrich sticks its head in the sand to hide what is out there. I'm saying tune out what you know is out there, since you don't need its loudness in your face all the time.

The lifeblood of network TV, most of cable, and much of "social" media and mass communication and marketing is *conflict*. Without conflict, there is no drama, and without drama, there is no sale (or viewership). Even comedy is full of conflict.

Money, of course, is at the root of it all.

Fear, greed, anger, violence, envy, hero worship, discontent—this is what is pumped into your heads daily—nonstop. These are destructive emotions. The theory is that this is what motivates you to either buy something or vote a certain way. And, it seems that we can't get away from it.

How can you enjoy what is around you—in the present moment—when you are texting, phoning, checking your email, or keyboarding all the time, and being bombarded with negative energy or things that you don't even want to consider?

When you subtract the wasted time, technical fowl ups, and poor quality of service in our "service" economy—is the net result productive for most of us? "Tech" has sure destroyed a lot of jobs, that's for sure. Why waste hours of our precious day—which may be our last—doing all this nonsense?

The point is, all this is adding to our anxiety and stress by introducing conflict and uncertainty that we cannot really manage or control. We're going too fast—*too much* information. Stress and anxiety interferes with our ability to lead healthy lives, and our sense of peace (which is the opposite of anxiety).

So, throw away that smart phone (or at least turn it off for a long while). Don't sit in front of the TV. Find a hobby, like painting in oils, writing, gardening, stained glass making, or who knows what—just do it. If you need your smart phone for work, fine. When that is done for the day, get rid of it.

We know that stress and anxiety generate or prolong bad habits.

Smoking, drinking alcohol, binge eating, chewing our nails—the list is endless.

Through the creativity of hobbies, limiting destructive conflict, and enjoying the *natural, quiet* moments in our lives in the *present* tense, we can better manage our stress and lead healthier lifestyles. Hopelessness and lack of control diminish, and with it anxiety, binge eating, and other had habits.

Take home lessons:

Give Mindfulness a try.

Find creative hobbies and try to eliminate the negative influences of too much harmful conflict in our lives.

Limit the intrusiveness of our "information" technology, and spend that time and resources on proper exercise and nutrition instead—and hobbies.

Chapter 10: Your Doctors and Care

Doctors need to have great skill and learn a lot to apply their trade to patients. With increased managed "care," "Obama-care," and the increasing use of physician and nurse "extenders," patients must acquire more "patient skills" as well.

Your time spent with your doctor, unless you want to pay a lot of cash for the visit yourself and not through insurance, is getting more limited all the time. Insurance companies will only pay the doctor a set amount, and that amount is constantly being whittled down. To survive economically, health providers are forced to "streamline" their service.

Therefore, you must make every minute with your physician count. Don't waste those minutes by asking questions about drugs that you don't need just because you heard them on TV. If you are overweight, ask her questions related to that.

How much am I overweight for my build, age, and height? Is this affecting my blood pressure? Are my labs normal, especially my blood sugars and cholesterol levels? If they are elevated—how serious is that? Am I at significantly increased risk for stroke or heart attack?

She will probably tell you anyway, but don't take it for granted.

Ask your doctor if they are trained and experienced in sports and exercise medicine. Many doctors have completed rotations in such areas during residency or medical school. Others specialize in this area as an adjunct to their practice, and take continuing medical education for such.

Your primary doctor should probably be a Board Certified Internist or Board Certified sub-specialist in a medicine subspecialty—such as endocrinology or geriatric medicine. A Board Certified Family Practice doctor is also a good choice, especially if they have specialized training or courses in Sports and Exercise Medicine. Board Certified Physical Medicine and Rehabilitation physicians, who are MD's with specialized training in physical functioning and sports medicine and pain management, can also be recommended.

Ask these doctors about any exercise program you are considering, including the one in this book. Ask him to set any physical limitations that may be in order based upon your exam, labs, medical record, and risk factors. Are there any pulse rate limits?

If possible, ask him to share specifics about the type of exercises they recommend, and perhaps even refer you to a trainer or physical therapist for special concerns. These concerns could be exercising with a bad knee, ways to reliably monitor your pulse during exercise, and what subjective factors to use in assessing exercise tolerance and intensity.

If your doctor is irritated with such questions or says he just doesn't offer guidance with exercise and dieting, nor has little training in that area, consider getting a new doctor. However, given today's medical practice landscape, that may be difficult. Your health plan may not allow you to choose so freely.

If so, then request a referral to a physical therapist for a specific medical problem surrounding your daily functioning. For instance, if you have a bad knee that is painful, you might mention that you may have trouble navigating stairs and curbs and need specific exercises and training from a physical therapist to ensure safety. For the over-fifty crowd especially, this is appropriate and invariably true.

Then, you can direct some of your exercise questions to your therapist, as long as your doctor has set the specific safety limitations based upon your medical record.

If you are new to physical fitness, over fifty, and have been sedentary most of your life, ask about special tests (such as a treadmill exercise stress test) to clear you for rigorous exercise *before* you start an exercise program. Insurance may not cover this, so if you have "risk factors" for heart attacks or strokes, that will help. For example, if you have anyone in your family who died of those disorders at a relatively young age, make that known to your doctor so she can document it.

It is very appropriate for you to be concerned about your safety during vigorous exercise.

If diabetes, strokes, or heart attacks do run in your family with any regularity, make sure your doctor is aware of that and puts that in the chart, especially if you have any symptoms that suggest dizziness, chest pains, visual disturbances, intermittent numbness in your body, or swallowing problems.

Give the doctor a clear and brief picture of your medical history to supplement what is in the chart.

Remember, he may not see you next time. It may be the "extender," so the information must be clear and concise enough to be transmitted into checked boxes that will be in the digital medical record (computerized records and all the inherent problems that go with it).

This may be what the physician's aid is reading on your next visit.

You might want to type out a paragraph summary of any important medical history along with a short list of your medications with dosages—and ask him to put it in your chart to supplement the computerized record, if possible. That way you're covered if the computer is down again.

When discussing your labs with your internist, make sure you ask her if she ran a "thyroid panel" on you. Thyroid problems, especially in patients over fifty, are common—especially in women. Usually the problem is a low functioning organ.

This means that your body is not producing enough thyroid hormone, and you may need supplementation. The internist (or preferably the endocrinologist if she refers you to one) follows a lab value called a TSH (thyroid stimulating hormone) to titrate the exact amount of thyroid hormone you should be taking.

This needs to be ample, but not too high.

In an exercise and dieting program, where you are trying to loose significant weight, ample thyroid supplementation is vital. You wouldn't expect a car to burn gasoline properly (and hence run efficiently) if the idle were so low that it constantly stalled.

You must have proper thyroid coverage. If you can, see a Board Certified endocrinologist.

Also, men—especially those over fifty— should have their free testosterone checked, since it may be very low. If so, this can cause lassitude, low libido, inadequate muscle tissue response to exercise, and fat burning and distribution issues.

These days, there are drugs to assist the "sleepy" target organ to produce more sex hormone, rather than injecting such a hormone directly into the bloodstream. There are risks. Ask your doctor about your free testosterone level.

Of course, women should consult their gynecologist also, where sex hormone issues are a bit more involved.

This brings into mind the whole "anti-aging" trend in medicine. Many doctors are specializing in this. However, some feel that the doctor practicing in this area should be Board Certified by the American Board of Medical Specialties in one of the internal medicine specialties, preferably endocrinology. They should also be experienced in dispensing such medicines, and have taken continuing medical education. Consult your internist, or ask for a referral to a Board Certified endocrinologist.

Actually, for most, intense exercise is the real fountain of youth.

If you snore, are having sleep problems that are serious enough to be interfering with your functioning, and you're overweight, make sure you inform your doctor about your insomnia. Enquire about a sleep program referral and a possible "overnight sleep study" (*sleep apnea, sleep study, sleep center, sleep medicine, disorders, body weight, brain activity and REM sleep*).

Many chiropractors have extensive training in sports medicine and physical rehabilitation, and, with your medical doctor, make a great adjunct to your pool of experts who can guide you in your diet and exercise program—and weight loss. Chiropractors are noted to be very service oriented.

They will spend time with you discussing your lifestyle changes, exercises, and physical limitations regarding exercise—especially neck and low back precautions. Make sure that your cardiovascular exercise preclusions, if any, are clearly set by your medical specialist first.

Make good use of all your providers.

Trainers, although not doctors, can be very helpful in your program as outlined in this book. This has been emphasized throughout. Try to find one that will work in tandem with your medical doctor or chiropractor to make the most out of these chapters.

We've touched upon psychological areas such as mindfulness, stress, anxiety, depression, and addiction as topics interrelated with weight control and exercise. *Body image* is also important.

Sometimes, how we look at ourselves is critically distorted. We think we are fat, but really are emaciated. We think we are thin, but really are obese. The mirror—but really our brain—lies to us. If this is an issue for you, you should seek a referral to an exercise psychologist (if the problem is minor), or to a psychiatrist if the distortion is major.

You must use your overworked doctor correctly, and that is *your* responsibility.

You must deal in the *real* world, and that world unfortunately is becoming more precarious for patients.

Be informed, be helpful, and most importantly be *nice*—she or he is trying to help you the best they can.

Take home points:

Proper levels of thyroid and other hormones are important to success in losing weight efficiently.

Use your doctor's time wisely, since it is limited. Make sure they have specific information about your risk for stroke, heart attack, sleep apnea, or medical disorders that will complicate your entry into gradual but rigorous exercise, dieting, and weight loss. Make sure they have the information necessary for an effective and focused medical record in the chart—which will be computerized and used (and added to) extensively by non-doctors.

Be aggressive and smart in pursuing referrals to other health services and professionals that will facilitate your safe use of this program. Intelligently discussing your risk factors with your doctor will assist him in documenting the need for such services. This is vital, if you want the health insurance to cover it, and not you! "Preventive medicine" is more recognized now, but resources are limited.

Internists and Family Practice doctors, endocrinologists, physical therapists, credentialed trainers, Physical Medicine and Rehabilitation doctors, dieticians, psychologists, psychiatrists, podiatrists, and chiropractors are all good sources of help for this book's program.

Chapter 11: Kiss; Keep it Simple Stupid

This program is simple and reproducible. Do *not* complicate it. Its beauty is that it can be routinely and cheaply followed, and results will ensue.

Keep it simple. You will work up to six hours of exercises per week in six months, plus a few hours per week preparing your meals.

"Calories In": Your mainstay will be the Orangutan Giant Wok and Vegetable Stewpot, and you'll be raiding those any time you're hungry during the next six months. Try to follow a meal timetable the best you can, and put a huge, hot portion in the proper container for your work at lunchtime or for mid-day snacks. Just keep it in your car. Try to eat your last meal no earlier than seven, and eat a few pieces of fruit or cooked egg whites if you want before bedtime as snacks. Taking a simple multiple-vitamin daily is fine.

Do *not* go hungry, and eat *big* portions, not small. Don't fuss with too much measuring or dirty dishes—it's not necessary. The more green and orange and red and yellow stuff you put in the pot or wok, the healthier the mixture, as opposed to white and brown and black (there seems to be a shortage of blue food in nature—too bad!).

"Calories Out": You need to work big muscle groups repetitively to burn big calories and achieve an adequate conditioning benefit.

This means primarily engaging your *butt* muscles—your gluts (quads too). There are only a few ways to do this efficiently, routinely, and safely, and the best (especially for the over forty crowd) are probably the reclined exercise bicycle with variable resistance controls (with proper positioning), and the inclined treadmill—walking at adequate steepness to ensure intensity. The first is safer.

Intensity is key. No intensity, little gain in terms of calorie burn and conditioning. There is also less endorphin high, which is important. Progressive resistive exercises, performed slowly with "cam" weights, are for most of us (especially mature folks) the most practical, safe, and efficient way to maintain and build strength in our major muscle groups, which augment work capacity and therefore potential for marginal increases in caloric burn during intense aerobic exercise. The muscle sculpting benefit, with weight reduction, also looks good, especially with proper hip (butt) weight exercises. The key is to concentrate and feel the pleasant *burn in the butt*— not pain! Again, intensity is key.

What could be simpler than the above? If you don't already belong, join a health club to see if you like this program. Give it at least three months. You must consult your doctor before you start, especially the more mature readers out there. You must consult the staff of the club to make sure you are doing the exercises safely and effectively.

Engage a trainer that you trust to help you.

After a month or so, if you like the program, consider buying the machines recommended in this book—but you must consult the proper credentialed heath professionals first to ensure safety. If you do buy them, you should retain your club membership if you can afford it (and again, have the sales person thoroughly ground you in the use of the machines).

It is money very well spent.

After you've completed six months of the program and have lost twenty-five to thirty pounds, consider staying on the modified version of the program (with occasional greater degrees of freedom in food choices), either to lose an additional thirty pounds, or just to help retain the progress you've already achieved. Keep on it as a plan for life. You can also tweak your favorite dishes to get more "calorie bang" out of the "buck" (more on that later).

If you do go for losing an additional thirty pounds, you will find—unlike other "diet" programs—the going gets much easier and fun. If so, you can make fitness a hobby and spend all the time you can afford doing it. But, it won't be *necessary* to make fitness your hobby.

Choose a few creative hobbies instead, and pull the plug on your smart phone and boob tube (at least for half the day).

This program will be with you for life.

I think you'll stick to it.

After all, you have to trust something, right? Why not . . . ok, enough all ready—I'll shut up!

Chapter 12: 12 Points; Dr. Blue's Day

Meet Dr. Sheila Blue. She is a forty-five year old radiologist, who lives in California and is divorced with two kids—both almost out of high school.

She is five foot three, and one hundred and forty-seven pounds, and of "medium" build. She has been exercising off and on for thirty years and has tried many diets. None of them resulted in lasting success.

She is attractive, but when she's dressed and in front of the mirror—she feels that she looks "frumpy." Her dress sizes are creeping up. She feels tired and finds her job stressful.

Sheila is very self-conscious about her weight, and therefore dates little.

Dr. Sheila Blue is a binge eater, and when she has a glass of wine, even the pipes in the refrigerator are not safe. She loves peanut butter, chocolate cake, and spaghetti—and refuses to do without them. She thinks that she exercises quite a lot, with two-mile walks around her neighborhood and lap swimming three times per week.

She never gets colds, and thinks that she is very healthy.

Since she's busy, the single radiologist doesn't have hobbies, and lately has been watching a lot of TV and cable while fooling around with her smart phone. It seems she is always being texted and called, mostly about junk. She's getting tired of it.

Finances are shaky, since expenses are high. She frets about bills, although she always seems to make ends meet at the end of the month.

Sheila feels that life is unfair. She is healthy and "fit," but has been dealt a bad hand—in that "her genetics" dictate that she will always look plump. At a party recently, someone got drunk and told her that she looked like a pumpkin in her new orange dress.

She went home and cried.

Sheila now sleeps poorly. She thinks it's because she frets about the future and her recent divorce too much, and future bills for college for her kids. Lately, she's been snoring (or so her kids say).

She wakes up in the middle of the night. In the morning, she doesn't feel refreshed, and sometimes her memory isn't up to snuff. Although it's mostly on the weekends, she is drinking too much wine too, sometimes a bottle a night. No one knows this, but she even takes an occasional "sleeping pill."

Dr. Blue recently visited her internist. Sheila had told him that her mother had died of a stroke at age sixty. Her medical history and physical exam were normal except that her doctor told her she could stand to lose twenty-five to thirty pounds, and her BP was a bit elevated at 150/90. Her thyroid level was also low.

Her labs came back abnormal.

Serum cholesterol level was 240, and her blood glucose level was 210. Her cardiogram looked fine. Her *current* thyroid hormone level was even lower than previous old labs indicated. Based upon her history the doctor suggested a referral to the sleep center and a pulmonologist.

Sheila wants to loose bulk—and pounds. The internist said that he would be glad to recommend a trainer. He also has a chiropractor he refers to that specializes in sports medicine.

Before she begins her diet and exercise program, the internist wants to schedule her for a treadmill exercise stress test to make sure she is sound from a cardiovascular standpoint.

The internist then told her that she has a mildly increased risk for stroke and heart attack and possibly even cancer, based upon her weight, labs, mildly elevated blood pressure, and family history. She needs to change her ways, and watch her salt intake.

She needs to lose thirty pounds and keep it off.

When the stress test result came back normal, her internist told her that she had no specific exercise preclusions from a medical standpoint, although she should start slow and use "common sense." Sheila looked online to browse "diet books."

She found a book with "orangutan" in the title, and since she loves apes, she decided to give it a try. After all, the book was short and the guy who wrote it is a physical medicine and rehabilitation specialist. She decided to download it on her Kindle through Amazon, the one she got for Christmas and hadn't yet used.

Dr. Sheila Blue visited the chiropractor and went over some of the exercises in the book with him. He demonstrated a few. She also called her internist to make sure that he was comfortable with the exercises and diet she was planning on doing.

Sheila liked the information in the book about "mindfulness," and performed a Google search to find out more. She also took up yoga and meditation. She strictly limited her smart phone use and turns off her TV set after dinnertime. She already has downloaded several books relating to concepts in the "orangutan" plan, reading them in her second Kindle (for audiobooks too). The ability to change the size of the text is key to her enjoyment, since small print gives her a headache. She has researched many topics this way. Reading's now a hobby.

Sheila had gone to Costco and purchased the recommended items. She prefers the Asian seasonings. She prepared her fist orangutan wok and stewpot with ease, and cooked the rice. She decided to put small squares of turkey breast into the pot. She loves her lunch container full of vegetables, and eats a huge portion while taking her half hour break at work. She concentrates on every bite of the vegetables.

She threw away the pie, the ice cream, and the loaf of bread in her refrigerator, along with the meat loaf. Often, she'll eat the boiled egg whites (with a little yolk) for snacks. She loves the fruit.

Dr. Blue purchased a membership at the local club, which is open twenty-four hours. She was instructed on the use of the treadmills (the wide version) and reclined exercise bicycle.

While using both, the trainer taught her postures and machine settings that helped her isolate her butt muscles.

She started with the treadmill at 4 degrees, 3.5 miles per hour, for ten minutes (including a short warm-up and cool- down). Before she started, she performed gentle stretches that her trainer showed her.

Sheila stuck to her program with the treadmill, but in the first six weeks saw little progress. She was still the same dress size, and that was very disconcerting. But, she *felt* better.

She gradually increased her incline degrees on the treadmill and length of time on the machine. She then gradually increased the speed to 3.8 miles per hour. Toward the end of the sessions, she started to feel a sense of elation and a "head rush."

By the time the third month ended, she was at an incline of 15 degrees, thirty minutes (with cool-down and warm-up), and 4 miles per hour, six days per week.

With a slight body and knee repositioning, and concentrating on her butt contractions, she could feel a prolonged burn and tightening. She loved the sweat and "rush" that she got.

Sheila was at first displeased with the meals in the program. "Is this it?" she would ask herself incredulously. "There must be more to it."

But, it was because there *wasn't* more to it that she stuck with it. It was so easy.

After four weeks, she started to enjoy the simple but rich taste of the vegetables more and more. She felt wonderful after she ate them. It simplified her life. She enjoyed the whole fruit treats an hour before bed. She let the kids eat what they wanted, and they could join with her in the meals later if they wished. They had their own lives.

Sheila also noticed that her food bill was cut in half (at least for her if not her kids). What she loved most is that she was never hungry but rather pleasantly full. She usually had a big portion of pot vegetables as a snack when she got home from work, then ate her dinner about seven. She never woke up hungry.

On the few binges she had, she ate from the pot, and it satisfied her.

Dr. Blue's internist started her on her thyroid medicine. She will see an endocrinologist for follow up on that problem.

She also found the sleep program referral very helpful. The cause of her snoring and insomnia and lassitude was indeed a mild sleep apnea. The sleep study confirmed this. This was found to be a "mechanical" problem related to her excess weight, and would probably resolve with weight reduction.

At the end of the tenth week, Sheila weighed herself and was very pleased to see a seventeen-pound weight reduction, along with a diminished dress size. At the end of the third month, she had lost twenty-two pounds.

Her butt was more rounded, firmer, and "felt much tighter." She started to look good in jeans—at a smaller size. She slept much better and felt more refreshed in the morning, with no more midnight awakenings.

Sheila found that at work she was more attentive, cheerful, and *looked* much better. At the end of six months, Dr. Sheila Blue had lost thirty-two pounds, dropped two sizes, and felt great.

She was less anxious, and could tolerate stressful situations with a lot more ease. She had taken up oil paining in the last two months, which enhanced her cool. Now she reads countless books on her Kindle, and is able to enjoy them and concentrate better. She now listens to audiobook painting lessons while painting.

When she revisited her internist, he was just as pleased as she was. Her labs, including blood sugars and cholesterol levels, were normal, and her blood pressure as 115/78.

In the last six months, she had nearly neutralized (except for the family history) her risk level for stroke and heart attack, and her cancer risk as well. Her sleep apnea, and all the ills that go with it, was virtually cured.

As far as continuing the orangutan program, she is on it for life. She discussed further weight reduction with her internist, and they felt it was unnecessary. She just wants to keep her loss.

She has all the opportunities to eat some of her old foods, but she doesn't feel the overwhelming compulsion to consume them as she had before. She feels calm and able to manage her life. She does not feel deprived. Some of her old goodies she found leaner substitutes for, such as ground lean turkey meatballs and spinach spaghetti with Prego Light Smart sauce instead of her old calorie blast.

She is very happy.

Life's wonderful bounty had returned to her, and she is pursuing her new hobbies with even more vitality and vigor. She now has a full *personal* life as well.

Sheila looks great, is even dating again, and was told that her butt "looks very well sculpted and yet supple." This was a reliable source.

How did that person know for sure?

Well . . . never mind.

Twelve major take home messages (put this on your refrigerator, next to the orangutan photo):

Cook your simple Orangutan vegetable stewpots and woks (don't complain just eat it). Always eat the food hot and eat slowly.

Buy your whole fruit as snacks and dessert. Use your eggs. Forget salads except when going out on free days later, they are too much work and the dressings can be monster calories and fat grams.

Burn your butt with the inclined trainer or reclined bicycle. Do it with adequate intensity to obtain benefit and gradually increase the challenge (incline and resistance) of your exercise, then time, the number of days per week, then speed. Get a club membership, and then buy your machines if you can.

Strengthen your major muscle groups with the progressive resistive exercises with limited (15) reps, until you achieve a mild burn—not pain. You must do this with sufficient intensity and SLOWLY to obtain benefit, or you are mostly wasting your time.

Do not weigh yourself until you have been on the program ten weeks, to avoid stress and pointless anxiety. Then, do it weekly.

You must consult your doctor *before* you start your exercise program to obtain medical clearance for physical exertion. For the over-fifty crowd or those with a history of medical issues, this is even more important.

Discuss with your doctor your specific risk for stroke and heat attack, and how much weight loss is necessary to help correct some of the factors that add to your risk. Make sure your thyroid level is sufficient to burn calories efficiently. If you have trouble sleeping, snore, and are overweight, discuss sleep apnea with your doctor, particularly if you are over forty. Check your free testosterone (men!).

Protect your joints from trauma. Strengthening exercises and weight loss are great ways to start. If you have a back or neck condition, seek physician guidance and be careful.

Most high blood pressure can be successfully treated with a thirty-pound weight loss. The sodium blasts from our processed foods complicate treatment, but the orangutan wok and vegetable stewpot can greatly help neutralize that problem. Eat it heartily.

Chemicals, additives, and toxins adulterate our food supplies, and navigating those hazards should be in your radar. Good washing of all your fresh vegetables is a practical way to start.

Ample thyroid replacement medication after expert testing, ideally from your Board Certified endocrinologist, is a must in any age group, but particularly in women over fifty. Unless this is corrected, *any* exercise and diet program will be less successful.

Stress and anxiety reduction is minimized through filtering out harmful noise and intense negative energy and conflict, and limiting your smart/cell phone usage, TV hours, and the texting and the ubiquitous email circus. Replacing that time with creative hobbies and *restful* relaxation is key. Mindfulness is a philosophical and psychological concept that may deserve your study. Depression, addiction, stress, and anxiety are interwoven and induce binge eating, illicit drugs (including alcohol), and poor sleep—all of which profoundly impact our weight control and general health.

Graduation

I know, I know, the food isn't fancy and the exercises simplistic to all you exercise buffs—but this book isn't written primarily for you. Its messages are directed mainly to the vast majority of middle aged women (and men) who *don't* have a history of being athletes and aren't even particularly interested in fitness—and are thirty to sixty pounds overweight.

These people just want to enjoy their lives more and hopefully dodge some serious diseases.

But—to the rest of you—this book can help you also.

So, quit griping and nitpicking about what is simplistic or subject to argument, and just get on with that part of it you like! Tweak it if you must.

It works.

It works in many slight variations.

But, you need to clear your rigorous exercise and diet first with your doctor, chiropractor, and trainer.

You will also be more informed about your general medical condition if you consult your doctors as you have been advised this book.

You will also be able to discuss your medical record more intelligently, assist with proper documentation in the chart, and focus on serious potential diseases that are impacted by your weight and condition.

This plan won't eat up your savings or your time either—so you'll have resources to use for your creative new hobbies (and to buy your machines)!

It won't introduce you to potentially harmful drugs or silly contraptions that you see by the hundreds on late TV (and for which billions are spent annually).

It will give you a blueprint to use for the rest of your life, while allowing occasional diversions. On your "free days," why not use your ingenuity and skill in experimentation to develop your own low fat and low calorie "mini-recipes" that are quick and don't dirty pots and dishes. This way, you can have bigger portions and less fat grams. Think of these recipes as functionally replacing certain favorite, fattening dishes, such as a big slice of apple pie or an ice cream sundae (for example, the Nabisco brand of low fat cinnamon graham cracker is a great "crust" for a healthy "pie." Add to each of four crackers a heaping spoonful of Simple Truth Organic brand fruit spread, and a tiny dab of butter, and you have yourself a great desert substitute (wash it down with half a glass of ice-cold skim milk!).

There are hundreds of such satisfying substitutes.

We have discussed anxiety, depression, and addiction, and focused on topics that you can explore further if you feel so inclined.

The harmful condition of sleep apnea is in your radar now, and you know what to do if you think you may suffer from it.

Bad habits, or alcohol and drug binging, can easily derail your weight and fitness program. It's wise to get a handle on those issues.

Sodium and salt ingestion was a big topic in this book, and now you have more information and tools to deal with it. The Giant Orangutan Wok and Giant Orangutan Vegetable Stewpot are natural, fresh, low salt solutions to your diet that are indispensable in tackling this very important issue (they will also keep you "regular" naturally!). Sodium control is nearly as challenging as weight control and fitness themselves.

The big bonus is, you may be able to add years to your life, and *quality* too, if you follow the basic precepts in this book.

Congratulations, you have now graduated from Orangutan Weight Control School.

Now that six months have passed since you have started on the program, and you are now using it for life (or an extra thirty pound loss first), I want you to go out to your favorite Halloween store (they are open all year) or costume shop.

I want you to buy an ape mask.

. . Yes, that's right, an *ape* mask.

Put on your best clothes.

Then, take your pen, and a little note about four-inches-square, and write on it in these words: "SAVE ME!"

Pin the note to your blouse or shirt.

Find the swankiest store in town. Prance around the store in your mask.

I hope you attract lots of attention.

I hope, if anyone asks you about the note (maybe the mask too!), you can tell them about the impending extinction of the Great Apes in Asia and Africa (You can tell them about the book too if you want!).

Tell them to join you in saving the apes.

These noble creatures are facing extinction if not more is done to protect them. Perhaps you can take up their cause at work, or sponsor a fundraiser.

If you have a local zoo, maybe partner with them to promote the preservation of our closest "ancestors," especially if they have a primate exhibit.

I pledge that five dollars out of every hundred of profit from this book or its derived formats (it will be on Audible audiobook and Kindle too) will be donated to an appropriate charity whose primary mission it is to save the apes.

Maybe you also can donate to an appropriate organization that is dedicated to the same goal.

Please, join with me in helping them to survive. They deserve to live. "They are just monkeys," you say. Compare their social history with ours, and their ability to harmonize with the planet, and it may be an open question as to which of the two of us is more intelligent—depending upon the definition.

One of my favorite movies of all time is the original *Planet of the Apes* with Charlton Heston—I never forgot the ending. Consider buying it on Amazon and play it.

Good luck to you, and happy and leaner trails.